PSYCHOSOCIAL DIMENSIONS OF CANCER

A NOTE FROM THE PUBLISHER

Cancer Nursing: Principles and Practice, Second Edition by Groenwald, Frogge, Goodman, and Yarbro is the best-selling text ever published for oncology nurses. Nurses around the world commonly refer to this landmark text as the "encyclopedia" of cancer nursing.

Over the years, oncology nurses have expressed a desire to have *Cancer Nursing* available in smaller, more specialized parts. Today, with the growing specialization within the oncology nursing field, this demand has increased.

In light of the tremendous demand, we are pleased to publish the individual parts from *Cancer Nursing*. All eight Parts are available in paperback format. (Parts VIII and IX have been combined).

In order to maximize the utility of the individual parts we have structured them as follows:

1. All parts have complete front matter (preface, foreword, and table of contents) from the main text. This helps the user understand how and where the individual part fits into the scope of the main text. In addition, the foreword by Vincent T. DeVita Jr., MD provides an interesting insight into the oncology field and should be read by all oncology nurses.
2. All parts have the complete index from the main text. This allows the user to identify additional topics available in *Cancer Nursing* and in the individual parts.
3. All parts maintain their page numbers from the main text. Therefore, the pages of the individual part will start on a page number consistent with the main text and not necessarily from page one.

Thank you for supporting our oncology nursing series.

PSYCHOSOCIAL DIMENSIONS OF CANCER

Part IV from
CANCER NURSING
Principles and Practice
Second Edition

EDITED BY

Susan L. Groenwald, RN, MS

Assistant Professor of Nursing—Complemental
Department of Medical Nursing
Rush University College of Nursing

Rush-Presbyterian-St. Luke's Medical Center
Chicago, Illinois

Michelle Goodman, RN, MS

Assistant Professor of Nursing
Rush University College of Nursing
Teacher / Practitioner
Department of Surgical Nursing
Section of Medical Oncology

Rush-Presbyterian-St. Luke's Medical Center
Chicago, Illinois

Margaret Hansen Frogge, RN, MS

Senior Vice President, Clinical Services
Coordinator, Community Cancer Program

Riverside Medical Center
Kankakee, Illinois

Connie Henke Yarbro, RN, BSN

Editor, *Seminars in Oncology Nursing*
Clinical Associate Professor
Department of Medicine
Division of Hematology / Oncology

University of Missouri—Columbia
Columbia, Missouri

JONES AND BARTLETT PUBLISHERS
BOSTON

Editorial, Sales, and Customer Service Offices
Jones and Bartlett Publishers
20 Park Plaza
Boston, MA 02116

ISBN   0-86720-303-X

The selection and dosage of drugs presented in this book are in accord with standards accepted at the time of publication. The authors and publisher have made every effort to provide accurate information. However, research, clinical practice, and government regulations often change the accepted standard in this field. Before administering any drug, the reader is advised to check the manufacturer's product information sheet for the most up-to-date recommendations on dosage, precautions, and contraindications. This is especially important in the case of drugs that are new or seldom used.

Printed in the United States of America
95 94 93 92 91   10 9 8 7 6 5 4 3 2 1

Katherine T. Alkire, RN, MN
Oncology Clinical Nurse Specialist
St. Luke's Regional Medical
    Center
Boise, ID

Barbara D. Blumberg, ScM
Director of Education
Komen Alliance Clinical Breast
    Center
Charles A. Sammons Cancer
    Center
Baylor University Medical Center
Dallas, TX

Joy H. Boarini, RN, MSN, CETN
Professional Education Manager
Hollister Incorporated
Libertyville, IL

Ann Rohman Booth, RN, BSN
Clinical Research Nurse
Hematology and Oncology
University of Arizona Cancer
    Center
Tucson, AZ

Jean K. Brown, RN, MS,
    PhD Cand.
University of Rochester
School of Nursing
Rochester, NY

Patricia Corcoran Buchsel, RN,
    BSN
Director, Outpatient Nursing
Fred Hutchinson Cancer
    Research Center
Seattle, WA

Candace Carter-Childs, RN, MS
AIDS Project Case Manager
Hospice of Marin
Marin County, CA
Assistant Clinical Professor
University of California
San Francisco, CA

Jane C. Clark, RN, MN, OCN
Oncology Clinical Nurse Specialist
Assistant Professor
Emory University
Atlanta, GA

Rebecca F. Cohen, RN, EdD,
    CPQA
Instructor, Community Health
School of Allied Health Profes-
    sions
Northern Illinois University
DeKalb, IL

Mary Barton Cook, RN, BSN,
    OCN
Director of Nursing
Oncology Program Coordinator
CPS Pharmaceutical Services
IV and Nutritional Services Divi-
    sion
Mountain View, CA

Vincent T. DeVita, Jr, MD
Physician-in-Chief
Memorial Sloan-Kettering Cancer
    Center
New York, NY

Kathy A. Dietz, RN, MA, MS
Nurse Clinician—Hematology
Memorial Sloan-Kettering Cancer
    Center
Associate
Columbia University School of
    Nursing
New York, NY

Joanne M. Disch, RN, PhD
Clinical Director
Department of Medical Nursing,
    Emergency Services and Dialy-
    sis
Hospital of the University of
    Pennsylvania
Assistant Professor of Nursing
University of Pennsylvania School
    of Nursing
Philadelphia, PA

Michele Girard Donehower, RN,
    MSN
Student, Nurse Practitioner Pro-
    gram
University of Maryland School of
    Nursing
Baltimore, MD

Constance T. Donovan, RN,
    MSN, FAAN
Oncology Clinical Nurse Specialist
Yale New Haven Hospital
Associate Clinical Professor
Yale University School of Nursing
New Haven, CT

Diane Scott Dorsett, RN, PhD,
    FAAN
Director
Comprehensive Support Services
    for Persons with Cancer
Associate Clinical Professor
University of California
San Francisco, CA

Susan Dudas, RN, MSN
Associate Professor
College of Nursing
University of Illinois at Chicago
Chicago, IL

Ellen Heid Elpern, RN, MSN
Clinical Nurse Specialist
Section of Pulmonary Medicine
Assistant Professor of Nursing
Rush University
Rush-Presbyterian-St. Luke's
    Medical Center
Chicago, IL

Dolores Esparza, RN, MS
President
Esparza Oncology Consultants,
    Inc.
San Antonio, TX

Betty Rolling Ferrell, RN, PhD, FAAN
Research Scientist, Nursing Research
City of Hope National Medical Center
Duarte, CA

Anne Marie Flaherty, RN, MS
Administrative Nurse Clinician
Adult Day Hospital
Memorial Sloan-Kettering Cancer Center
New York, NY

Arlene E. Fleck, RN, MNEd
Clinical Cancer Research Coordinator
Cancer Prevention Center
Kelsey-Seybold Foundation
Houston, TX

Marilyn Frank-Stromborg, RN, EdD, Nurse Practitioner, FAAN
Coordinator
Oncology Clinical Specialist Program
Professor
School of Nursing
Northern Illinois University
DeKalb, IL

Margaret Hansen Frogge, RN, MS
Senior Vice President, Clinical Services
Coordinator, Community Cancer Program
Riverside Medical Center
Kankakee, IL

Gayling Gee, RN, MS
Director, Outpatient Nursing
San Francisco General Hospital
Assistant Clinical Professor
School of Nursing
University of California
San Francisco, CA

Barbara Holmes Gobel, RN, MS
Oncology Clinical Nurse Specialist
Lake Forest Hospital
Faculty, Complemental
Rush University College of Nursing
Chicago, IL

Michelle Goodman, RN, MS
Oncology Clinical Nurse Specialist
Section of Medical Oncology
Assistant Professor of Nursing
Rush University
Rush-Presbyterian-St. Luke's Medical Center
Chicago, IL

Marcia M. Grant, RN, DNSc, OCN
Director of Nursing Research and Education
City of Hope National Medical Center
Duarte, CA

Susan L. Groenwald, RN, MS
Oncology Nurse Consultant
Assistant Professor of Nursing— Complemental
Rush University College of Nursing
Chicago, IL

Shirley M. Gullo, RN, MSN, OCN
Oncology Nurse
The Cleveland Clinic Foundation
Cleveland, OH

Patricia Hakius, RN, MSN
Cancer Care Consultant
Doctoral Student
University of San Diego
San Diego, CA

Nancy E. Harte, RN, MS
Oncology Clinical Nurse Specialist
Section of Medical Oncology
Rush-Presbyterian-St. Luke's Medical Center
Instructor
Rush University College of Nursing
Chicago, IL

Laura J. Hilderley, RN, MS
Oncology Clinical Nurse Specialist
Private Practice of Philip G. Maddock, MD
Radiation Oncology
Warwick, RI

Barbara Hoffman, JD
Private Consultant
Cancer Survivorship and Discrimination
Princeton, NJ

Catherine M. Hogan, RN, MN, OCN
Oncology Clinical Nurse Specialist
Department of Hematology/ Oncology
University of Michigan
Ann Arbor, MI

Susan Molloy Hubbard, RN, BA
Director
International Cancer Information Center
National Cancer Institute
Bethesda, MD

Patricia F. Jassak, RN, MS, CS
Oncology Clinical Nurse Specialist
Foster G. McGaw Hospital
Loyola University of Chicago
Chicago, IL

Judith (Judi) L. Bond Johnson, RN, PhD
Nursing Director
North Memorial Medical Center
Minneapolis, MN

Paula R. Klemm, RN, DNSc Cand.
Nursing Instructor II
The Johns Hopkins Oncology Center
Baltimore, MD

Linda U. Krebs, RN, MS, OCN
Oncology Nursing Program Leader
University of Colorado Cancer Center
Denver, CO

Charles E. Kupchella, PhD
Dean
Ogden College of Science, Technology and Health
Western Kentucky University
Bowling Green, KY

Jennifer M. Lang-Kummer, RN, MS
Oncology Clinical Nurse Specialist
Beaumont County Hospital
Washington, NC

Susan Leigh, RN, BSN
Cancer Survivorship Consultant
Tucson, AZ

Julena M. Lind, RN, MN
Executive Director
Center for Health Information,
    Education and Research
California Medical Center
Adjunct Assistant Professor of
    Nursing
University of Southern California
Los Angeles, CA

Ada M. Lindsey, RN, PhD
Dean and Professor
School of Nursing
University of California
Los Angeles, CA

Lois J. Loescher, RN, MS
Research Specialist
Program Coordinator
Cancer Prevention and Control
University of Arizona Cancer
    Center
Tucson, AZ

Alice J. Longman, RN, EdD
Associate Professor
College of Nursing
University of Arizona
Tucson, AZ

Jean McNicholas Lydon, RN, MS
Oncology Clinical Nurse Specialist
Department of Therapeutic
    Radiology
Rush-Presbyterian-St. Luke's
    Medical Center
Chicago, IL

Mary B. Maxwell, RN, C, PhD
Oncology Clinical Nurse Specialist
Nurse Practitioner
Veterans' Administration Medical
    Center
Portland, OR

Mary Dee McEvoy, RN, PhD
Robert Wood Johnson Clinical
    Nurse Scholar
Hematology/Oncology Section
Division of Nursing
Hospital of the University of
    Pennsylvania
Philadelphia, PA

Rose F. McGee, RN, PhD
Professor
American Cancer Society
    Professor of Oncology Nursing
Emory University
Atlanta, GA

Deborah B. McGuire, RN, PhD
Assistant Professor
The Johns Hopkins University
    School of Nursing
Director of Nursing Research
The Johns Hopkins Oncology
    Center
Baltimore, MD

Joan C. McNally, RN, MSN
Executive Director
Michigan Cancer Foundation
    Services, Inc.
Detroit, MI

Nancy Miller, RN, MS
Assistant Director of Testing
    Services
National Council of State Boards
    of Nursing, Inc.
Chicago, IL

Ida Marie (Ki) Moore, RN, DNS
Assistant Professor
College of Nursing
University of Arizona
Tucson, AZ

Theresa A. Moran, RN, MS
Oncology/AIDS Clinical Nurse
    Specialist
Oncology/AIDS Clinic
San Francisco General Hospital
Assistant Clinical Professor
School of Nursing
University of California
San Francisco, CA

Marian E. Morra, MA
Assistant Director
Yale University Comprehensive
    Cancer Center
New Haven, CT

Lillian M. Nail, RN, PhD
Assistant Professor
University of Rochester School of
    Nursing
Clinician II
University of Rochester Cancer
    Center
Rochester, NY

Susie Lee Nakao, RN, MN
Nurse Manager
Clinical Research Center
Los Angeles County
University of Southern California
Los Angeles, CA

Denise Oleske, RN, DPH
Research Associate
Department of Health Systems
    Management
Department of Preventive
    Medicine
Rush-Presbyterian-St. Luke's
    Medical Center
Assistant Professor
College of Health Systems
    Management
Rush University
Chicago, IL

Sharon Saldin O'Mary, RN, MN
Home Care Coordinator
Stevens Cancer Center
Scripps Memorial Hospital
LaJolla, CA

Edith O'Neil-Page, RN, BSN
Nursing Supervisor
The Kenneth Norris Jr. Hospital
    and Research Institute
Los Angeles, CA

Diane M. Otte, RN, MS, ET
Administrative Director—Cancer
    Program
St. Luke's Hospital Cancer Center
Davenport, IA

Geraldine V. Padilla, PhD
Associate Professor
Associate Dean for Research
School of Nursing
University of California
Los Angeles, CA

Mary Pazdur, RN, MS, OCN
Head Nurse
Discharge Planning
The University of Texas
M.D. Anderson Cancer Center
Houston, TX

Patricia A. Piasecki, RN, MS
Joint Practice
Section of Orthopedic Oncology
Rush-Presbyterian-St. Luke's
    Medical Center
Chicago, IL

Sandra Purl, RN, MS, OCN
Oncology Clinical Nurse Specialist
Section of Medical Oncology
Rush-Presbyterian-St. Luke's
    Medical Center
Instructor
Rush University College of
    Nursing
Chicago, IL

Kathy Ruccione, RN, MPH
Division of Hematology Oncology
Children's Hospital of Los Angeles
Los Angeles, CA

Beth Savela, RN, BSN
Graduate Student
Oncology Clinical Specialist
Program
School of Nursing
Northern Illinois University
DeKalb, IL

Vivian R. Sheidler, RN, MS
Clinical Nurse Specialist in
Neuro-Oncology
The Johns Hopkins Oncology
Center
Baltimore, MD

Joy Stair, RN, MS
Education Specialist
Department of Nursing Education, Quality and Research
Catherine McAuley Health Center
Ann Arbor, MI

Debra K. Sullivan, RD, MS
Research Specialist in Nutrition
Center for Handicapped Children
University of Illinois Hospital
Chicago, IL

Debra J. Szeluga, RD, PhD
Assistant Professor of Clinical
Nutrition
Assistant Professor of Medicine
Section of Medical Oncology
Co-Director
Nutrition Consultation Service
Rush University
Rush-Presbyterian-St. Luke's
Medical Center
Chicago, IL

Mary Taverna, RN
Executive Director
Hospice of Marin
Marin County, CA

Claudette G. Varricchio, RN,
DSN, OCN
Associate Professor
Medical-Surgical Nursing
Niehoff School of Nursing
Loyola University of Chicago
Chicago, IL

JoAnn Wegmann, RN, PhD
Assistant Administrator
Director of Nursing Services
Poway Community Hospital
Poway, CA

Deborah Welch-McCaffrey, RN,
MSN, OCN
Oncology Clinical Nurse Specialist
Good Samaritan Cancer Center
Phoenix, AZ

Debra Wujcik, RN, MSN, OCN
Oncology Clinical Nurse Specialist
Oncology/Hematology
Vanderbilt University Medical
Center
Adjunct Instructor of Nursing
Vanderbilt University School of
Nursing
Nashville, TN

Connie Henke Yarbro, RN, BSN
Clinical Associate Professor
Department of Medicine
University of Missouri-Columbia
Editor, *Seminars in Oncology
Nursing*
Columbia, MO

J. W. Yarbro, MD, PhD
Professor of Medicine
Director of Hematology and
Medical Oncology
University of Missouri-Columbia
Columbia, MO

FOREWORD

The pace of development in the cancer field and the gratifying assumption of a greater role for nurses in the delivery of cancer care dictates the need for freshness in a modern nursing text on cancer. The second edition of this text provides the opportunity to maintain that freshness. It also provides the opportunity to reflect on where we have been and where we are going. Much of the progress taking place can be described as occurring in two overlapping waves; a breathtaking wave of new technology, developed as a consequence of the biologic revolution, lapping at a wave of significant improvements in technology in existence before 1971. Nineteen seventy-one is a good benchmark year; the key event that year was the passage of the National Cancer Act. The vision of the architects of that Act was prescient. The resources supplied by the US Congress fueled the biologic revolution that is now affecting all of medicine. Before then we had little appreciation of the mechanism of uncontrolled growth we call cancer and how the cell machinery was damaged in the process of carcinogenesis. We knew early diagnosis was useful but not why, and while we had refined methods to control primary tumors with surgery and radiotherapy, more than 65% of the patients died of their disease as a result of micrometastases already present at the time of diagnosis, not included in surgical or radiation treatment fields. To overcome this problem, surgery and radiotherapy had become radicalized, and often mutilating, in an attempt to widen their impact on the illusive cancer cell, which was envisioned as spreading by contiguous involvement of adjacent tissue before entering the blood stream. The use of systemic therapy, concomitant with local treatment, was controversial and of unproven value. Attempts at prevention were almost nonexistent.

In other words, cancer was like a black box. We could remove it or destroy it, when we could identify it; we could examine it, we could measure it, we could weigh it, but we could not out-think it because we could not effectively look inside the cell itself. The biologic revolution wrought by the Cancer Act provided the tools of molecular biology that changed all that.

Now the cancer cell is like a blue print; not only is the machinery of the cancer process exposed for examination and manipulation, but also in this exposure we have uncovered important information in developmental biol-ogy—the essence of life itself. We now know that cell growth is controlled by a series of growth regulating genes that operate in a biologic cascade from recessive suppressor genes to dominant genes we know as proto-oncogenes in normal tissue and as oncogenes in cancer tissue, of which there are now more than 40 identified. These genes code for growth factors, their receptors, membrane signal transducing proteins, protein kinases, and DNA binding proteins, all important in signal transmission, which in turn is the way multicellular organisms maintain order in their community of cells. While these genes are involved in normal growth and development, mother nature has wisely provided a means for suppressing their expression in mature organisms since their continued operation would be dangerous. Similarly, the metastatic process is no longer thought to be a random phenomenon tied only to tumor growth but has been found to be an aberration of the process of cell migration in normal development and, like the growth controlling function of oncogenes, subject to manipulation by molecular methods. Cancer can result from damage to any of several of the steps in this genetic cascade. Inherited loss or damage of an allele of a recessive suppressor gene appears to lead to a release of the cascade of oncogenes and uncontrolled expression. Damage to a dominant oncogene can lead to escape from control by suppressor genes. Overproduction of a normal or abnormal protein product of an oncogene can occur due to failure of the cell to respond to "off" signals. The startling advances in molecular technology make it possible to isolate and manipulate the products of these genes with ease and use them as diagnostic and therapeutic targets. This was the promise of the cancer program and this is the payoff.

This new wave is, however, just now reaching the level of practical use. For example, in diagnosis, molecular probes and the extraordinarily sensitive polymerase chain reaction can be used to diagnose gene rearrangements to determine cell lineage in malignancies of lymphoid origin, and specific sequences at break points of nonrandom chromosome translocations can be used to diagnose solid tumors. The polymerase chain reaction can be used as a tool to monitor the effects of treatment by detecting one residual malignant cell out of a million normal cells. A molecular approach to treatment also is surfacing in the form of antisense message compounds, chemically stabilized pieces of DNA complementary for, and inhibitory to, the message strand of the DNA of an operational gene or the message of specific target genes such as oncogenes. An extension of this approach will be the use of analogs of the recently identified products of suppressor genes to attempt to bring the oncogene cascade under control. A crest of this new wave of technology in treatment has reached the clinic in the practical application of the colony-stimulating factors produced through DNA recombinant technology, which is already influencing the use of chemotherapy, and the recombinant-produced interleukins and interferons, which have already produced useful antitumor effects by themselves.

Perhaps the most important and often overlooked implication of the biologic revolution is in its potential to allow meaningful approaches to cancer prevention. One of the main roadblocks to testing new ways to prevent cancer has been the identification of groups of high-risk populations small enough to allow prospective prevention trials to proceed at reasonable costs and with a reasonable prospect of answering important questions in the lifetime of the involved investigators. Genetic analysis of common tumors such as colon, breast, and lung cancers following on the heels of the first work on the identification of deletion of suppressor genes in the rare tumor retinoblastoma indicates that deletions of suppressor genes are common and likely to be tumor specific. These new approaches, when applied to the population at large, should allow us to identify individuals at high risk for getting common cancers. Then and only then can we accurately determine if the many interesting leads in prevention identified in the vast number of epidemiologic studies supported by the cancer program over the last two decades can truly be exploited to prevent common cancers.

This then is the new wave. A simultaneous wave of advancement in existing technology of a more practical nature has occurred in cancer management. The emergence of high-speed computers converted roentgenographic diagnosis and staging from plain film and linear tomography to computerized tomography and made magnetic resonance imaging an indispensable tool. Older, less precise, more morbid methods of diagnosis and staging have slowly, and appropriately, fallen into disuse. In 1971, we had just become aware that drugs could cure some types of advanced cancer, and the exploration of adjuvant chemotherapy had just begun. Now adjuvant drug treatments have proven beneficial in breast, colon, rectal, ovarian, head and neck, bladder, and pediatric tumors and in some kinds of lung cancer and bone and soft tissue sarcoma. Chemotherapy has quietly become the primary treatment for all stages of some types of lymphomas and for some stages of some types of head and neck cancers and bladder cancers. We also have developed a greater appreciation of the reason for treatment failure. A form of multiple drug resistance has been described in common tumors, derived from tissue exposed to the environment, that affects drugs derived from natural sources like some of our best antitumor antibiotics. We are just now begin-

ning to design protocols to circumvent multidrug resistance. The use of bone marrow transplantation to support high doses of chemotherapy has made us acutely aware of past treatment failures due to inadequate dosing that can now be overcome with concomitant use of colony-stimulating factors to promote more rapid recovery of bone marrows. New radiotherapy equipment, coupled with computerized tomography treatment planning, has made radiotherapy less morbid and more acceptable as an alternative to radical surgery.

As a consequence of all this, combined modality treatment is no longer what it was in the early 1970s. It no longer means doing the standard radical surgical procedures, adding the standard extensive and toxic radiation therapy fields, and later the standard drug combination, but instead initial treatment is being offered with a precise design based on the capability of each modality in controlling local tumor and metastases while minimizing toxicity. In other words, cancer management has become a complex medical jigsaw puzzle administered by dedicated professionals, many of whom are nurse practitioners, and almost unnoticed, has become far less morbid. Since cancer treatment is still far too morbid, this latter change has been difficult for many to appreciate. However, those of us who have seen both ends of the spectrum over the past two decades have a greater appreciation of the change in morbidity of treatment than a newcomer. Nowhere is this change more evident than in breast cancer where 15 years ago a radical mastectomy followed by postoperative radiation cured a handful of patients, while leaving the few survivors with the morbid effects of a denuded chest wall and a swollen nonfunctional arm. Now survival is improved with specifically tailored local and systemic treatment with fewer side effects and excellent cosmetic results. Fifteen years ago nausea and vomiting, pain, and marrow suppression were largely uncontrollable side effects, and now all can be managed to a great degree.

Unlike the new wave of advances in molecular biology, which remains to be widely implemented before it will have an impact on cancer mortality, the improvement in current technology has already had an impact on national statistics. In 1971, the relative survival rate for all cancers combined was barely 36%; it has increased to 49% in the last available data ending in 1985. Declines in national mortality, formerly only noted in children under the age of 15, are now apparent in all age groups up to age 65, and if one excludes lung cancer, a largely preventable disease, a decline in national mortality is noted all the way up to age 85.

The challenge before us is to smooth the transition of these successive waves of progress into medical practice. It has never been easy because one must recognize them as they exist, separate and distinct bodies of knowledge, each affecting medical practice in different ways, but waves that will eventually summate. Their combined impact gives us the means to effect a significant reduction in cancer mortality by the year 2000. Successful reduction in cancer mortality, however, depends on a cooperative partnership between the medical profession and the public to use modern information to prevent cancer and to implement newly developed treatment rapidly and effectively nationwide. Aside from lagging support for cancer research, which threatens the momentum of change, the machinery in place to do all this is hampered by outdated regulations, unimaginative reimbursement policies, medical territoriality, and unwarranted pessimism about the prospects for controlling cancer in our lifetime. The prospects have never been better but, as the framers of the National Cancer Act knew, nonscientific reasons and failure of all of us to think about controlling cancer on a national scale are major deterrents to success. Nurses reading this text should keep this in mind because they will play an increasingly important role in the next decade in bridging the various medical specialty interests and the delivery of the new cancer care.

VINCENT T. DeVITA, JR, MD

Physician-in-Chief
Memorial Sloan-Kettering Cancer Center
1275 York Avenue
New York, New York 10021

PREFACE TO THE SECOND EDITION

Our goal in the second edition of *Cancer Nursing: Principles and Practice* is to provide the reader with the most comprehensive information about cancer nursing available in the 1990s. Each of the original 44 chapters in the first edition was thoroughly reviewed and updated. Twenty-five new content areas were added, including Relation of the Immune System to Cancer, Cancer Risk and Assessment, Biotherapy, Bone Marrow Transplantation, AIDS-Related Malignancies, Late Effects of Cancer Treatment, Psychosocial Dimensions: Issues in Survivorship, Sexual and Reproductive Dysfunction, Oncologic Emergencies, Delivery Systems of Cancer Care, Economics of Cancer, Teaching Strategies: The Public, and Teaching Strategies: The Patient. This edition contains 60 comprehensive chapters representing the contributions of over 75 recognized oncology nursing experts.

The exponential increase in information about oncogenes resulting from a massive research effort has provided a greater understanding of the nature of carcinogenesis. This improved understanding is reflected in this second edition and will continue to have a significant impact on the nature of clinical care. Even with this research effort and greater understanding of the nature of carcinogenesis, however, it is unlikely that a magic cure or vaccine for cancer will be available in the near future. There will continue to emerge new approaches to early diagnosis of cancer, new techniques to treat cancer, new measures to ameliorate distressing manifestations of cancer and its treatment, and new approaches to improve the quality of life for cancer survivors. Cancer nurses are integral to these developments. It is to these nurses that this text is dedicated.

The editors wish to gratefully acknowledge the tremendous effort of the contributors who enthusiastically shared their knowledge and expertise and gave their time and energy to this endeavor. We wish to especially acknowledge our husbands Keith, Jim, Larry, and John for their assistance, support, and patience during this mammouth project.

The editors have developed this text to be a comprehensive resource for nurses who provide or manage care for patients in the home, hospital, or community, who teach patients and nurses, and who conduct research to find better approaches to patient care—all of whom contribute to our steady gains in providing quality care to individuals with cancer.

SUSAN L. GROENWALD
MARGARET HANSEN FROGGE
MICHELLE GOODMAN
CONNIE HENKE YARBRO

PREFACE TO THE FIRST EDITION

This text is one I always wished to have. As a graduate student of oncology nursing, and later as an oncology clinical nurse specialist and educator at Rush-Presbyterian St. Luke's Medical Center, I became frustrated by the dearth of texts written at the level of the oncology graduate student or oncology nurse specialist. Oncology nursing texts lack the depth and breadth of scientific information that I believe is an essential element in the armamentarium of the professional nurse; medical literature, while it contains the necessary scientific information, lacks application of scientific principles to the nursing care arena.

In this text, the contributors and I committed ourselves to presenting the reader with the most comprehensive information about oncology nursing available, including relevant science and clinical practice content that addresses both the whys and hows of oncology nursing practice. All chapters cite original published research as the scientific foundation for the application of these findings to clinical practice. All students of oncology nursing—beginning or advanced—will find this book valuable as a text and as a reference for clinical practice.

The disease of cancer in the adult is approached from many angles to address the complex learning needs of the oncology nurse specialist. Part I includes cancer epidemiology and deals with individual and societal attitudes toward cancer and the impact of attitudes on health behaviors. Part II provides the foundation of scientific information about the malignant cell on which all subsequent chapters are built. Concepts such as carcinogenesis, oncogenesis, metastasis, invasion, and contact inhibition are included in Part II, and thorough attention is given to changes that occur in a normal cell and its behavior as it transforms to a malignant cell.

In Part III, the psychosocial dimensions of cancer are approached according to critical phases through which patients, families, and caregivers may pass as they cope with the stressors induced by cancer. Part IV presents a conceptual approach to the most common manifestations of cancer and their effects on the individual with cancer. Each chapter includes pathophysiology, assessment, and medical and nursing therapies. Part V describes each of the major cancer treatment methods, their uses, adverse effects, and nursing care considerations for individuals receiving cancer therapy. Included in this part is a chapter on unproven methods of treatment. Part VI is a comprehensive review of most of the major cancers by body system and the problems experienced by people who live with cancer. (Information pertaining to pediatric malignancies and nursing care of the child with cancer has been omitted. Although pediatric oncology is a critical area of interest for many nurses, it could not be covered in sufficient depth within this text.) Part VII presents continuing-care options for the individual living with the problems imposed by cancer. Part VIII analyzes several issues relevant to the oncology nurse: consumerism, ethics, cancer nursing education, and cancer nursing research. Part IX, which lists oncology resources of many types, is a handy reference tool.

Some of the information presented in this text is out of date even as it is written because of ever-expanding knowledge about cancer and its treatment. As Dr. Vincent DeVita remarked at his swearing-in as Director of the National Cancer Institute (*The Cancer Letter*, 1980:4), "What we now know of the cancerous process and what we do to prevent, diagnose, and treat it will be outmoded and radically different by the end of the 80s." This book is our best effort to put down in writing the science and art of cancer nursing in the 1980s.

SUSAN L. GROENWALD

The Jones and Bartlett Series in Nursing

Basic Steps in Planning Nursing Research, Third Edition
Brink/Wood

Bone Marrow Transplantation
Whedon

Cancer Chemotherapy: A Nursing Process Approach
Burke et al.

Cancer Nursing: Principles and Practice, Second Edition
Groenwald et al.

Chronic Illness: Impact and Intervention, Second Edition
Lubkin

A Clinical Manual for Nursing Assistants
McClelland/Kaspar

Clinical Nursing Procedures
Belland/Wells

Comprehensive Maternity Nursing, Second Edition
Auvenshine/Enriquez

Critical Elements for Nursing Preoperative Practice
Fairchild

Cross Cultural Perspectives in Medical Ethics: Readings
Veatch

Drugs and Society, Second Edition
Witters/Venturelli

Emergency Care of Children
Thompson

First Aid and Emergency Care Workbook
Thygerson

Fundamentals of Nursing with Clinical Procedures, Second Edition
Sundberg

1991-1992 Handbook of Intravenous Medications
Nentwich

Health and Wellness, Third Edition
Edlin/Golanty

Health Assessment in Nursing Practice, Second Edition
Grimes/Burns

Healthy People 2000
U.S. Department of Health & Human Services

Human and Anatomy and Physiology Coloring Workbook and Study Guide
Anderson

Human Development: A Life-Span Approach, Third Edition
Frieberg

Intravenous Therapy
Nentwich

Introduction to the Health Professions
Stanfield

Management and Leadership for Nurse Managers
Swansburg

Management of Spinal Cord Injury, Second Edition
Zejdlik

Medical Ethics
Veatch

Medical Terminology: Principles and Practices
Stanfield

Mental Health and Psychiatric Nursing
Davies/Janosik

The Nation's Health, Third Edition
Lee/Estes

Nursing Assessment, A Multidimensional Approach, Second Edition
Bellack/Bamford

Nursing Diagnosis Care Plans for Diagnosis-Related Groups
Neal/Paquette/Mirch

Nursing Management of Children
Servonsky/Opas

Nursing Research: A Quantitative and Qualitative Approach
Roberts/Burke

Nutrition and Diet Therapy: Self-Instructional Modules
Stanfield

Oncogenes
Cooper

Personal Health Choices
Smith/Smith

A Practical Guide to Breastfeeding
Riordan

Psychiatric Mental Health Nursing, Second Edition
Janosik/Davies

Writing a Successful Grant Application, Second Edition
Reif-Lehrer

CONTENTS

PART IV

PSYCHOSOCIAL DIMENSIONS OF CANCER

Chapter 16

Overview of Psychosocial Dimensions

Rose F. McGee, RN, PhD

INTRODUCTION

The focus of the psychosocial dimension of cancer care is the unique needs of the individual at risk for or with cancer and the social groups affected by that individual. Each individual brings to the cancer experience unique personality traits and a personal socialization pattern different from all others. Understanding the uniqueness of the individual is achieved only through study of the commonalities of the "personality and social psychological"[1] aspects of illness.

To separate the dimensions of health care into physical and psychosocial is artificial, yet it serves pragmatic purposes in narrowing the scope of the discussion. In fact, a whole body of literature exists on the study of psychosocial variables as a risk factor in carcinogenesis. Lickiss[2] noted that reviews of cancer research in the nineteenth century indicated that "while tissue and cellular changes were the characteristic phenomena of cancer, both inherent susceptibility and extrinsic influences played a part in the genesis of these phenomena—by mechanisms unknown" (p. 297). More recently, the study of psychosocial factors as independent variables has been focused on the study of the immune and endocrine systems as mechanisms of causation.[3] Thus the study of psychosocial variables as causative is an evolving area of study in oncology that may provide future clues to prevention.

In the meantime, professional commitment to quality of care and to holistic care has resulted in a focus on psychosocial aspects of illness as outcome variables of the cancer experience. Empirically, the prevalence of psychosocial distress in response to a diagnosis of cancer has been found to range from a rare occurrence to as high as 90% of all patients.[4] The burgeoning number of studies on variables that maximize self-actualization and minimize psychosocial distress offers new understanding about the meaning of the diagnosis of cancer and response patterns of individuals and groups to the actual or perceived threat.

The purpose of this chapter is to address the ubiquitous threat of cancer and to discuss the use of psychosocial resources to manage responses. To choose one theoretical orientation would be reductionistic, and to discuss the breadth of psychosocial theories is prohibitive; therefore, the chapter is of necessity an overview of selected concepts derived from the theoretical, empirical, and experiential body of knowledge of the psychosocial aspects of cancer and cancer care. A basic assumption of the following discussion is that psychosocial responses to the cancer experience are determined by the characteristics of cancer, the person with or at risk for cancer, and the social system of significance to the individual.

CANCER: THE UBIQUITOUS THREAT

The only certainty in oncology is that cancer is an actual or potential threat to all humans. Statistically, one in three persons and three of every four families will experience cancer. But statistics apply to groups and serve a minimal purpose in assessing individual risks. A small percentage of the population can personalize the risk further because of genetic predisposition to cancer, but for the majority, cancer risks are the product of unmeasurable, cumulative life-style and environmental exposure. Therefore to live in the current physical and psychosocial environment is to be at risk for cancer. The particular risk will vary with age, geographic location, and life-style choices, but no individual or social sector is exempt.

The threat or diagnosis of cancer can be characterized as follows:

1. The meaning to the individual is unique.
2. The disease and treatment are marked by uncertainty.
3. Cancer is a chronic illness.
4. Cancer results in a changed identity.
5. Cancer affects the entire social system of the person involved.

Cancer Is a Unique Experience

The stigma of cancer has been traced historically by Cassileth[5] from the naming of the disease by Hippocrates as *karkinos*, which means crab, to the seventeenth and eighteenth century notion that cancer was contagious, which led to the use of the word "tumor" or other euphemisms to minimize isolation of persons with the diagnosis. During the nineteenth century, "tumors" were classified as benign or malignant, and further pathologic delineation lead to the contemporary understanding of cancer as a composite of many diseases. Cassileth[5] described the last 50 years as an era in which cancer is no longer met with fearful retreat in Western cultures but is met with a more frontier-type spirit, as evidenced by the "war on cancer." Nevertheless, the stigma of cancer continues to exist with respect to social and individual perceptions. Insurance cancellations, job and military discrimination, and problems with reintegration into the school and workplace are manifestations of the persistent social stigma of cancer.

The prevailing Western view of cancer is that cancer is a treatable disease. The resulting societal expectation is that the individual will accept the diagnosis, seek care, and comply with a fighting spirit.[5] Nevertheless, to the individual, cancer has been described as the "ultimate existential crisis."[6] For most persons, cancer is among the most feared of all diseases.[7] Reasons listed for the fear of cancer include the occurrence without warning, uncontrollable spreading of the disease, incurability beyond a certain point, association with pain and discomfort, social and professional attitudes of hopelessness, difficulty of diagnosis, mutilative treatment, unknown causation, and the fact that cooperation with treatment does not necessarily lead to successful outcomes.[8]

In Western societies, health is a value and illness is experienced as a barrier to the achievement of valued goals; therefore the perceived threat of cancer includes a subjective evaluation of the threat to health in general and the threat of cancer in particular. Smith[9] provided a multidimensional and hierarchial description of health that is useful in studying the impact of cancer on health in general. According to Smith, perceptions of health range from the most primitive level of absence of pathology, to disruption of role functioning, to ability to adapt, to the highest level, which is self-actualization. Because of the problems of diagnosis and of determining spread or recurrence of disease, each dimension of health may be disrupted. A perceived absence of pathology with respect to cancer is never certain among both the general population and persons previously diagnosed with cancer; both ascribed and achieved roles are temporarily or permanently disrupted; the ability to adapt may be exceeded by the demands of the illness; and safety and survival needs may supercede self-actualization goals.

Cognitive appraisal[10] of the personal meaning of cancer and the impact on life goals determine the meaning of cancer to the individual. Knowledge of and past experiences with the disease are but two variables that influence psychosocial and behavioral responses. According to the health belief model,[11] necessary conditions for preventive or curative care include some knowledge of the disease, perceived vulnerability, motivation to seek help, and perceived benefits that exceed barriers to action.

In summary, the threat of cancer is a unique process determined by cognitive appraisal of the situation. Threat appraisal is subjective and includes evaluation of the adequacy of resources to deal with the perceived situation. Cohen and Lazarus[12] summarized patterns of cancer threat perceptions as follows:

1. Fear of dying
2. Changes in body integrity and comfort
3. Changes in self-concept and disruption of future plans
4. Inability to maintain emotional equilibrium
5. Lack of fulfillment of social roles and activities
6. Inability to adapt to new physical and social environments

Disease and Treatment Are Marked by Uncertainty

Experiential knowledge of delays in diagnosis, short illness trajectories, unpredictable prognoses, and early death in apparently healthy individuals compound the uncertainties associated with the cancer diagnosis and prognosis. Mishel[13] defined uncertainty as the "inability to determine the meaning of illness-related events" (p. 225). Uncertainty results from the inability to structure the meaning of illness-related stimuli to form a cognitive schema for the illness events perceived. Stimuli consist of symptom patterns, event familiarity, and event congruence between the expected and experienced patterns. The degree to which the specific malignancy fits the criteria for uncertainty outlined by Mishel is determined by the degree of:

1. Ambiguity concerning the state of the illness
2. The complexity of treatment and the system of care
3. Information held about the diagnosis and seriousness
4. Predictability of the course and prognosis.

Although these criteria are useful in determining the predicted degree of uncertainty of the specific cancer diagnosis, uncertainty is not inherent in the situation but is a perception of the individual. The cognitive capacity of the individual and perceived resources influence the outcomes of this appraisal process.[13] According to crisis theorists, the perception may be interpreted as a danger or as an opportunity for growth.

Cancer Is a Chronic Illness

Much has been written about the chronicity of cancer. Of significance with respect to management of psychosocial responses is the fact that simple crisis resolution models are not sufficient to address the scope of problems encountered with cancer. Mages and Mendelsohn[14] noted that people with cancer are confronted with a continuing series of stressors rather than with a single, time-limited crisis. The treatment is complex, often extended, and may cause irreparable damage to physical, mental, or social functioning. Patients identify the lifelong fear of recurrence as one of the most disruptive aspects of the illness.

Application of stress management theory to the cancer experience makes the health care professional attentive to the fact that the initial adaptive responses used by patients may be outmoded as the disease process and treatment change.[14] For example, denial may be adaptive in the early stages of the disease as a defense mechanism, allowing the individual to assimilate the impact of the illness in manageable increments of awareness. By the same token, persistent denial may block motivation of adaptive health behavior in later stages of the illness. Likewise, the preoccupation with self that is characteristic during diagnosis and recurrence may initiate problem-solving coping behaviors during these stressful events but may alienate the person's social and professional network if persistent.

A further implication of the usefulness of stress theory in understanding psychosocial responses is the consideration of the effect of cumulative stressors on the ability to adapt. Individuals come to the cancer experience with a history of stress responses. The individual who has been unsuccessful in resolving past stress situations, who is dealing with a number of stressors simultaneously, and who perceives minimal social support in the situation is at higher risk for psychosocial distress.

The Cancer Experience Results in a Changed Identity

The majority of individuals who encounter cancer report permanent changes in self-perception and future orientation. Weisman and Worden[15] used the Inventory of Current Concerns to accrue empirical data on changes in emotional responses and interpretation, in reactions to others and to one's immediate world, and in thoughts of life, death, and survival. The concept of "existential plight" was used to refer to this grouping of perceptions of self.

Some changes in identity are socially imposed, while others are internal in origin. Evans,[16] in describing a personal experience with cancer, related a vivid description of the interactional effects on identity:

> There I was. I had cancer—the big "C". . . . The initial period of discovering my cancer caused the most trauma with both family and friends. . . . I could not cope with that look in their eyes. I did not want their sympathetic glances, their hushed tones. I had not changed inside. I was still the same person. Yet suddenly I seemed to have become different; I had become a cancer victim, losing my personal identity at home and in the hospital. I tried to retain a normal life. . . . It was then that I decided a personal survival plan would help and support me. [The doctors] were great. They just listened. I just hoped that I had enough strength to fight long enough for my life. Then the waiting period. Another form of purgatory—to regain normality while waiting to see if the cure will be effective. I was fortunate to receive the constant support of my family, friends, doctors, and nurses. My role was to find the inner strength and determination to fight back. I hope if I was [sic] ever put to the test again I would be able to fight back—I know now I would try. Life is far more precious to me now (pp. 17-18).

Adaptive and defense mechanisms are means the individual uses to cope with the conflicts between the physiological, psychological and sociocultural demands of cancer. Repression, projection, reaction formation, situation avoidance, and transference have been observed in cancer patients coping with changes in identity inflicted by the diagnosis and treatment.[17]

The specific culture of the individual shapes the view of health in terms of the range of normal, cause and effect perceptions, and the language to describe deviations from normal. For example, in a culture in which life expectancy is short, cancer may be a less meaningful threat than in a culture in which the chronic diseases of aging are the leading causes of death.[18]

Finally, the culture, through socialization, shapes the more enduring aspects of the attitudes, beliefs, and values that constitute one's personality and that provide continuity in the reordering of the meaning of life and of one's relationship to a higher being. Cancer can challenge lifelong values and beliefs and may result in changed cognitive, affective, and behavioral responses.[18] Affective responses identified as occurring most frequently among cancer patients are anxiety and depression. No one response, per se, is either adaptive or maladaptive. The appropriateness of the response to the psychosocially constructed reality of the situation and adaptability of the social network in acquiring new patterns of response, as indicated, determine the adaptive potential of the specific response.

Cancer Affects the Social System of the Individual

Psychosocial responses may be categorized as a complex interaction of cognitive, affective, behavioral, and physical components. For example, a common cognitive response of patients and families is the "why me" phenomenon and a resultant search to make sense of a senseless situation. Causal attributions tend to cluster into the categories of self-blame and projection.[19] The cognitive search for causation may influence affective responses positively by dispelling some of the anxiety associated with the diagnosis or negatively by leading to self-doubt and hostility toward others. The behavioral response of continuously "telling one's story" may, in turn, lead to social rejection and further enhance physical feelings of distress.

Within the social milieu, the family may deal affectively with the problem of uncertain causation by blaming the patient and thus absolve personal guilt, while less intimate significant others or health care professionals may maintain cognitive beliefs in a "just world" by blaming the patient as well.[20] Thus a vicious cycle may emerge in which the person is held responsible for the illness by self or others, and the potential for psychosocial distress is heightened, especially if the disease is unrelenting or recurrent.

The level of perceived social support is a variable that is viewed as a buffer to the effects of stress on the health of the individual.[21] Postulated mechanisms of the buffering effect of perceived social support include diminishing the level of the perceived stress of the situation, facilitating coping effectiveness, and lessening the reactions of the individual to the stressors.[22]

THE SEARCH FOR PSYCHOSOCIAL RESOURCES

The search for psychosocial resources to deal with the actual or potential threat of cancer is generally initiated in terms of self-appraisal and can be conceptualized as expanding spheres to significant others and, finally, to members of the health care professions. Orem,[23] in emphasizing the self-care concept, heightened the awareness of the professional with respect to the fact that the initial help-seeking behaviors expand outward from the individual to the professional; likewise, the return to health should be manifest by the professional's returning the responsibility for health care to the family and ultimately to the patient. Fostering individual control, anticipatory socialization, and early discharge and rehabilitative planning are a few of the techniques that foster achievement of these goals.

In general, the primary objective of nursing intervention is to foster the coping responses of patients, significant others, and the health care team. According to stress theorists, coping may be emotion focused or problem-solving focused. Examples of emotion-focused interventions include fostering emotional expression through active listening; creating constructive release of affective responses through play therapy, music, or humor; fostering understanding of the impact of personal responses on others through role playing; and providing individual or group testing and counseling to facilitate insight into emotional needs and response patterns. Problem-solving interventions may include information giving on the subjective, environmental, and temporal features of diagnostic and treatment processes; anticipatory socialization to expected life stressors and processes, such as loss and grief; individual and group teaching based on assessment of learning needs; identification of resource information and personnel; and referral for more specialized or intensive therapy.

The taxonomy of nursing diagnoses developed in a series of National Conferences for Classification of Nursing Diagnosis (NANDA) reflects the commitment of the profession to addressing both patient and family responses to illness and treatment. Research findings that 65% to 75% of health care is provided by the patient or the family[24] and that the spouse is the primary mental health caregiver[25] attest to the appropriateness of nursing diagnoses specific to the individual and the family.

Finally, these diagnoses illustrate the fact that psychosocial responses include both the potential for distress and for growth. Nursing intervention to achieve the latter has been studied extensively, but methodologic problems and the complexity of human behavior hinder accumulation of definitive data on the relative effectiveness of each intervention. A recent review by Johnson and Lauver[26] of the theoretical and empirical relationships between preparatory information giving and coping with stressful treatment experiences is an example of the accrual of theoretical and empirical data that reflects both the progress and limitations in establishing the database needed to increase nursing effectiveness in dealing with the psychosocial aspects of cancer care.

CONCLUSION

The following two chapters provide models of more specific nursing approaches to the study of selected psychosocial responses to the actual or potential diagnosis of cancer. The focus of Chapter 17 is responses of the individual, and Chapter 18 addresses the interactional responses of the person and the social system. The final chapter in this section, Chapter 19, combines the responses of the person and the social network with respect to survivorship.

REFERENCES

1. Cooper C: The psychological precursors of cancer, in Cooper C (ed): Psychosocial Stress and Cancer. New York, John Wiley & Sons, 1984, pp 21-33.
2. Lickiss JN: The growing edge: Psychosocial aspects of cancer. Med J Aust 1:297-302, 1980.
3. Greer S: Psychological enquiry: A contribution to cancer research. J Psychol Med 9:81-89, 1979.
4. Farber JM, Weinerman BH, Kuypers JA: Psychosocial distress in oncology outpatients. J Psychosoc Oncol 2:109-118, 1984.
5. Cassileth BR: The evolution of oncology as a sociomedical phenomenon, in Cassileth BR (ed): The Cancer Patient: Social and Medical Aspects of Care. Philadelphia, Lea & Febiger, 1979, pp 3-16.
6. Brohn P: The Bristol Programme. London, Century Paperbacks, 1987.
7. Cox T: Stress: A psychophysiological approach to cancer, in Cooper CL (ed): Psychosocial Stress and Cancer. New York, John Wiley & Sons, 1984, pp 149-169.
8. Clark RL: Psychological reactions of patients and health professionals to cancer, in Cullen JW, Fox BH, Isom RN (eds): Cancer: The Behavioral Dimensions, New York, Raven Press, 1976, pp 1-10.
9. Smith JA: The idea of health: A philosophical inquiry. Adv Nurs Sci 3:43-50, 1981.
10. Folkman S, Schaefer C, Lazarus RS: Cognitive processes as mediators of stress and coping, in Hamilton V, Warburton DM (eds): Human Stress and Cognition. Chichester, England, John Wiley & Sons, 1979, pp 265-298.
11. Becker M, Haefner DP, Kasl SV, et al: Selected psychosocial models and correlates of individual health related behaviors. Med Care 15:27-46, 1977.
12. Cohen F, Lazarus RS: Coping with the stresses of illness, in Cohen F, Adler NE (eds): Health Psychology: A Handbook. San Francisco, Jossey-Bass, 1979, pp 217-254.
13. Mishel MH: Uncertainty in illness. Image: J Nurs Schol 20:225-232, 1988.
14. Mages NL, Mendelsohn GA: Effects of cancer on patient's lives: A psychological approach, in Cohen F, Adler NE (eds): Health Psychology: A Handbook. San Francisco, Jossey-Bass, 1979, pp 255-284.
15. Weisman AD, Worden JW: The existential plight in cancer: Significance of the first 100 days. Int J Psychiatr Med 7:1-5, 1976/1977.
16. Evans J: The cancer experience—a patient's view, in Pritchard AP (ed): Cancer Nursing: A Revolution in Care, Proceedings of the Fifth International Conference on Cancer Nursing. London, England, Macmillan Press, 1989, pp 17-18.
17. Westbrook MT, Viney LL: Psychological reactions to the onset of chronic illness. Soc Sci Med 16:899-905, 1982.
18. Haney CA: Psychosocial factors in the management of patients with cancer, in Cooper CL (ed): Psychosocial Stress and Cancer. New York, John Wiley & Sons, 1984, pp 201-227.
19. Bard MT: The price of survival for cancer victims, in Strauss AL (ed): Where Medicine Fails (ed 3). New Brunswick, NJ, Transaction Books, 1979, pp 225-236.
20. Lerner MJ: The desire for justice and reactions to victims, in Macaulay J, Berkowitz L (eds): Altruism and Helping Behavior. New York, Academic Press, 1970, pp 205-229.
21. Northouse LL: Social support in patients' and husbands' adjustment to breast cancer. Nurs Res 37:91-95, 1988.
22. House JS: Work, Stress and Social Support. Reading, Mass, Addison-Wesley, 1981.
23. Orem DE: Nursing: Concepts of Practice. New York, McGraw-Hill, 1985.
24. Levin L, Katz A, Hoist E: Self Care: Lay Initiatives in Health. New York, Prodist, 1976.
25. Oberst MT, James RH: Going home: Patient and spouse adjustment following cancer surgery. Topics Clin Nurs 7:46-57, 1985.
26. Johnson JE, Lauver DR: Alternative explanations in coping with stressful experiences associated with physical illness. Adv Nurs Sci 11:39-52, 1989.

Chapter 17

Psychosocial Dimensions: The Patient

Jane Clark, RN, MN, OCN

INTRODUCTION

Psychosocial responses to cancer are influenced by factors that create the perceived reality of cancer for the individual. The reality of the cancer experience is complex and uncertain and results in psychosocial responses that are dynamic, nonlinear, and nonhierarchial and that vary in severity. The complex intrapersonal and interpersonal reactions to the cancer experience mandate that health care professionals share a common concern and maintain a high index of suspicion for the occurrence of dysfunctional psychosocial responses. Focusing on systematic and continuous assessment for signs and symptoms of psychosocial responses, identification of dysfunctional responses, development of interdisciplinary interventions to facilitate adaptive psychosocial responses, and evaluation of the effectiveness and efficiency of selected interventions to meet identified needs can improve both the quantity and quality of survival for people with cancer.

What is the basis of psychosocial care in oncology? Historically, clinical case studies of individuals and groups experiencing cancer were used to identify the unique psychosocial responses to cancer, to describe the types of coping patterns among persons with cancer, and to guide health care professionals in assisting the person with cancer to adapt to the diagnosis, the demands of treatment, and the demands of living with a cancer diagnosis. Yet just as significant variability exists in physiologic responses to cancer of different sites as well as within the same site, the variability of psychosocial responses is multiplied by the fact that each individual brings his or her values, beliefs, attitudes, personality, resources, and coping patterns to the cancer experience.

Efforts of health care professionals to understand the unique psychosocial responses of persons with cancer have been enhanced through qualitative studies of the relationship of selected psychosocial variables to:

1. Physiologic factors, such as site of cancer, histology, grade, stage of disease, or treatment modality
2. Care settings, including primary, secondary, and tertiary care hospitals, outpatient clinics, and the home
3. Temporal elements of the disease trajectory, ranging from screening to diagnosis, primary treatment, recurrence or relapse, death, or long-term survival
4. Developmental stage of the individual, with emphasis on the responses of children and older adults

Yet the findings from qualitative studies often yielded conflicting results. Thus, health care professionals began to examine conceptual and theoretical inconsistencies of both clinical and empirical data. Recently researchers have focused on developing clarity and specificity in describing the psychosocial responses of persons with cancer. The development of instruments with acceptable reliability and validity estimates among persons with cancer, expansion of research methodologies to include qualitative methods, and development of advanced statistical modeling procedures to study the interaction of psychosocial responses both as dependent and independent variables have contributed to understanding complex psychosocial relationships.

The focus of this chapter is the psychosocial responses that are of high incidence among persons with cancer. Responses selected include anxiety, depression, hopelessness, and altered sexual health. An operational definition of each response has been developed. Selected research and clinical instruments to measure the response are described and a review of representative research articles addressing the incidence and relationship of the response to the cancer experience is presented. Finally, areas for future nursing research are suggested.

ANXIETY

Anxiety has been described, with depression, as the most common psychosocial reaction experienced by persons with cancer. However, limited data exist on the occurrence and patterns of anxiety in persons with cancer. Often associated with transitions in the course of the disease or treatment, anxiety is described as a recurring response, varying in levels of intensity throughout the cancer experience.

Operational Definition

Operationally, anxiety can be defined as follows:

- An individual exists with the ability to respond affectively to changes in the environment.

- The individual perceives certain beliefs, values, and conditions essential to a secure existence.

- The individual experiences a nonspecific internal or external stimulus that is perceived as a threat to the secure existence.

- *The individual responds to the perceived threat affectively with an increased level of arousal associated with vague, unpleasant, and uneasy feelings defined as anxiety.*

Measurement Instrument: State-Trait Anxiety Inventory

The instrument used most commonly to measure anxiety among persons with cancer is the State-Trait Anxiety Inventory (STAI).[1] The STAI consists of two scales, the A-trait and A-state. Subjects are asked to respond to 20 items (A-state) on a 4-point scale (not at all, somewhat, moderately so, and very much so). Responses are summed to measure how the subject feels at a particular moment. Scores indicate the level of transitory anxiety characterized by feelings of apprehension, tension, and autonomic nervous system–induced symptoms: nervousness, worry, and apprehension.

The trait inventory is designed to measure general level of arousal and predict anxiety proneness. Subjects are asked to respond to 20 items (A-trait) on a 4-point scale (almost never, sometimes, often, and almost always). Again, responses are summed to measure disposition to respond to a stressful situation with varying levels of A-state intensity and the degree to which presenting stimuli are perceived as dangerous or threatening. Scores range from 20 to 80 for each scale, with a higher score representing higher levels of anxiety.

Reliability estimates for the STAI have been reported in the alpha coefficient range of .83 to .92. Construct validity has been reported as point biserial ranges of .60 to .73 and alpha ranges of .83 to .94. Concurrent validity has been established with the Taylor Manifest Anxiety Scale ($r = .79$ to .83) and the Affect Adjective Checklist ($r = .51$ to .52). In addition, construct validity with the known groups technique has been established.[1]

Patterns of Occurrence

The occurrence of anxiety as a response to diagnosis and treatment of cancer was described in the literature by Lucente and Fleck,[2] who compared levels of anxiety between patients hospitalized with a diagnosis of cancer and with a nonmalignant condition. Findings indicated greater levels of anxiety in the group with a diagnosis of cancer. Similar findings have been reported by other researchers.[3,4]

Anxiety is increased at diagnosis and remains elevated in varying levels throughout the course of treatment regardless of treatment modality or setting. Surgery as a treatment modality in general elicits an anxiety response, yet when the surgery is for cancer, the response may be more severe. Morris and Royle[5] reported preoperative and postoperative levels of clinical anxiety among 20 patients with early breast cancer given a choice of surgery (simple mastectomy or wide excision and radiotherapy) and 10 patients not given a choice. Findings indicated that a significantly higher percentage of patients not offered a choice of surgery were clinically anxious preoperatively when compared with those patients given a choice ($p < .05$). For those patients offered a choice, no significant differences in clinical anxiety were found between those who had a simple mastectomy and those who had a wide excision and radiotherapy or between patients having surgery for benign breast disease ($n = 31$) and general surgical patients ($n = 20$).[5]

Oberst and Scott[6] reported no differences in anxiety scores among a group of patients with genitourinary cancer treated surgically with and without a resulting ostomy at five time periods from predischarge up to 180 days after discharge. Repeated measures ANOVA indicated that the pattern of anxiety scores were essentially linear with a significant time effect ($F(3,114) = 8.834$, $p < .0001$).[6]

To describe the emotional impact of surgical treatment

for breast cancer within the first year after surgery, Gottschalk and Hoigaard-Martin[7] analyzed data collected from a collaborative study group supported by the National Cancer Institute. At 1 to 3 months after surgery, 118 women who had a unilateral mastectomy for stage I or II breast cancer had significantly higher mean death, mutilation, and total anxiety scores as measured by the Gottschalk-Gleser Content Analysis Scale than did 64 women who had a biopsy for benign breast disease, 69 women who had a cholecystectomy, and 78 women who had not had a major surgical intervention. However, significant reductions in mean mutilation, shame, and total anxiety scores ($p < .01$) were reported in the mastectomy group 10 to 12 months after surgery.[7]

Similar patterns of anxiety responses appear in the literature concerning radiation therapy as a treatment modality. In a study of 181 patients receiving external radiation therapy for cancer, Irwin et al[8] found that all patients, male and female, exhibited higher anxiety scores than nonpatient norms before treatment. Yet higher anxiety scores were reported among female versus male patients before initiation of treatment, 1 week after treatment was completed, and 2 months after completion of therapy. Patients in general reported significantly higher anxiety during rather than after treatment.[8]

In another study, anxiety was examined among patients ($N = 45$) receiving external radiation therapy for cancer.[9] A pattern of anxiety responses emerged. Patients with lower anxiety scores (STAI) before treatment exhibited significantly higher A-state scores after treatment; patients with moderate anxiety scores exhibited little change in A-state scores; and patients with high anxiety scores exhibited a significant decrease in A-state scores after treatment. No such patterns of change were found for A-trait scores among any group, supporting the hypothesis that changes in scores were related to situational factors rather than personality factors.[9]

Andersen et al[10] studied anxiety, as measured by the STAI, among 19 patients with gynecologic cancers receiving intracavitary radiation. A-state scores ranged in the 74th to 95th percentiles for all patients. As the time for treatment neared, anxiety increased for patients in both the low- and high-anxiety groups. When treatment was completed, high-anxiety patients had significantly lower A-state scores, while the low-anxiety patient group scores remained unchanged, indicating residual anxiety.

Anxiety related to chemotherapy and associated side effects has been implicated in the decision of patients either to reject treatment or to withdraw before completing the recommended therapy.[11] In a study of 78 stage II patients with breast cancer receiving adjuvant chemotherapy, anxiety was reported in 97% of the subjects, yet the levels of anxiety were represented by low scores, indicating mild distress.

Cassileth et al[12] administered the STAI to 378 patients with cancer and 379 matched relatives. Mean anxiety scores among the patient group (37.2) were similar to scores among other physically ill patient groups yet were lower than scores among patients who were being treated for depression. Of note was the trend for state and trait anxiety scores to increase among patients under follow-up care, active treatment, and palliative care, respectively.

In a sample of 60 men cured of Hodgkin's disease, Cella et al[13] studied the occurrence of persistent anticipatory nausea, vomiting, and anxiety after chemotherapy. Data generated from a semistructured interview revealed that 80% of the subjects who had completed chemotherapy at least 6 months before the study complained of anxiety when reminded of treatment.

In summary, increased levels of anxiety have been associated with a diagnosis of cancer. Patients treated with surgery, radiation therapy, and chemotherapy have also reported mild or moderate levels of anxiety. Yet anxiety at minimal or moderate levels may be motivating for the patient.

Impact of Anxiety on Patient Outcomes

Although increased levels of anxiety among persons with cancer have been documented, few researchers have studied the impact of increased anxiety on patient outcomes. Scott[4] studied the relationship of anxiety, critical thinking, and information processing during and after breast biopsy. Anxiety levels (STAI scores) among the 85 patients studied were extremely high and above group norms for acutely ill psychiatric patients. Women with high anxiety scores were found to have positively correlated critical thinking ability (Watson-Glaser Critical Thinking Appraisal) scores. In addition, critical thinking was substantially reduced at hospitalization when compared with 6 to 8 weeks after discharge.

Carey and Burish[14] studied the impact of anxiety as a predictor of behavioral therapy outcomes for 72 patients receiving chemotherapy. Findings indicated that pretreatment anxiety was associated with treatment outcome. Patients with low anxiety had significantly greater reduction in diastolic blood pressure, self-reported anxiety, and depression when compared with patients with moderate and high anxiety. However, pretreatment anxiety levels were not related to nausea levels.

Therefore, beginning empirical data indicate that anxiety is associated with selected patient outcomes. The strength and direction of the relationships between anxiety and selected psychosocial intervening and outcome variables remains to be defined.

Assessment Criteria

Anxiety has been recognized as an accepted nursing diagnosis category by the North American Nursing Diagnosis Association (NANDA).[15] As such, a preliminary definition, possible etiologies, and subjective and objective defining characteristics have been developed (Table 17-1).[15] Efforts have centered on developing specific criteria for deriving the diagnostic statement, yet the required clustering of signs and symptoms critical to the diagnosis are unclear. In addition, the criteria for fear and anxiety are remarkably similar except for the ability of the

patient to identify the source of threat. Defining characteristics for anxiety include "fear"; defining characteristics of anticipatory anxiety include the designation of a "future/impending event perceived as a threat"; and contradiction exists over whether the consequences of the threat or the threat itself is the unspecified stimulus.

Consequently, the reliability and validity of the defining characteristics to predict the occurrence of anxiety are questioned. Thus, validation of the diagnosis with the perceptions of the patient is mandatory. Additional clinical research is needed to test the NANDA recommendations for definition and diagnostic criteria of anxiety. Critical characteristics to differentiate motivational versus dysfunctional anxiety also must be distinguished.

Nursing Interventions

Interventions are based on helping the patient to recognize the spectrum of manifestations of anxiety, to determine if the patient desires to do anything about the response, and to activate coping strategies to control anxiety levels.[16] Validation of observed manifestations of anxiety provides an opportunity for the patient to acknowledge or deny the presence of those manifestations and to prioritize the most disturbing responses. Although the manifestations may be classified by health care professionals as disturbing, the patient may perceive the level of anxiety experienced as positive and reject intervention.

However, if the patient expresses a desire to reduce the anxiety, the nurse has an opportunity to help the patient identify the threat, learn to modify responses to the stimuli, and channel the responses constructively. Based on the principles and assumptions of cognitive theory, the nurse may begin by exploring perceived patient concerns and helping the patient evaluate the concerns within the reality of the situation. Often the interventions of exploration and evaluation will result in the ability of the patient to focus on the threat or to appraise the stimuli in a different way, thus reducing anxiety.

Since the etiology of anxiety is defined as being nonspecific, interventions may focus on treating the symptoms by activating previously effective coping strategies or on teaching new strategies to control the anxiety. Each patient brings to the cancer experience a history of previous coping strategies that have been effective and ineffective in managing anxiety. The nurse has the opportunity to help the patient identify those strategies (Table 17-2)[17] used in the present milieu and evaluate the effectiveness of the strategies in reducing anxiety. For patients who desire to learn new strategies, the nurse may offer information through formal and informal education programs, assistance in problem solving through counseling, role modeling with anxiety-reducing techniques such as relaxation training or music therapy, or referral to support groups within the care institution and the community.

Few studies have been conducted among patients with cancer to determine the effectiveness of independent nursing interventions in reducing anxiety, yet available data indicate potential benefits for education programs,

TABLE 17-1 Nursing Diagnoses That Address Anxiety

Nursing Diagnosis	Definition	Defining Characteristics
Anxiety	Vague, uneasy feeling, the source of which is often nonspecific or unknown to the individual	Verbalizes apprehension, uncertainty, fear, distress, worry, verbalizes painful and persistent feelings of increased helplessness, inadequacy, regret, expresses concern (change in life events), fear of unspecified consequences, overexcited, rattled, jittery, scared, restlessness, focus on self, insomnia, increased perspiration, wariness, glancing about, poor eye contact, familial tension, voice quivering, increased tension, foot shuffling, hand and arm movements, trembling, hand tremor, shakiness
Mild Anxiety	Increased level of arousal associated with expectation of a threat (unfocused) to the self or significant relationships	Verbalizes feelings of increased arousal and concern, increased questioning, restlessness, increased awareness, attending, mild restlessness
Moderate Anxiety	Increased level of arousal associated with expectation of a threat (unfocused) to the self or significant relationships	Expressed feelings of unfocused apprehension, nervousness, or concern, verbalized expectation of danger, voice tremors, pitch changes, restlessness, increased rate of verbalization, pacing, hand tremor, increased muscle tension, narrowing focus of attention, diaphoresis, increased heart rate, respiratory rate, sleep or eating disturbances
Severe Anxiety (Panic)	Increased level of arousal associated with expectation of a threat to the self or significant relationships	Expressed feelings of unfocused, severe dread, apprehension, concern, or nervousness, inappropriate verbalization or absence of verbalizations, purposeless activity or immobilization, perceptual focus scattered, fixed, or inability to focus on reality, increased heart rate, hyperventilation, diaphoresis, increased muscle tension, dilated pupils, pallor
Anticipatory Anxiety	Increased level of arousal associated with a perceived future threat (unfocused) to the self or significant relationships	Indicators of anxiety (See Anxiety), future impending event perceived as a threat to physical or psychosocial self (unfocused)

Source: Gordon M: Manual of Nursing Diagnosis. New York, McGraw-Hill, 1987.

TABLE 17-2 Approach and Avoidance Coping Strategies

Approach Strategies	Avoidance Strategies
Information seeking	Denial of emotion
Participation in religious activities	Minimization of symptoms
	Social isolation
Distraction	Passive acceptance
Expression of emotion and feeling	Sleeping
Positive thinking	Substance abuse
Conservation of energy	Avoidance of decision making
Maintenance of independence	Blame others
Maintenance of control	Excessive dependency
Goal setting	

Source: Adapted from Miller JF: Coping with Chronic Illness: Overcoming Powerlessness. Philadelphia, FA Davis, 1983.

relaxation training, music therapy, and support groups. The following empirical studies are representative of the nursing literature with respect to the potential benefits of such interventions.

Johnson[18] reported on the effects of a patient education course on persons with a chronic illness. Fifty-two subjects were selected randomly from the patients with a first or recurrent diagnosis of cancer within a 12-month period. Preintervention measures of state anxiety (STAI), meaningfulness in life, and knowledge were obtained. Based on preintervention scores and demographic variables, subjects were paired. One subject from each pair was assigned randomly to the treatment group. Subjects in the treatment group attended eight educational sessions over a 4-week period. Content for the sessions included learning about the disease, managing daily health problems, communication, feeling good about oneself, living within physical limitations, and community resources. The experimental group had statistically significant lower anxiety scores than the control group.

Cotanch and Strum[19] reported on the effects of progressive muscle relaxation (PMR) on anxiety, nausea, and vomiting associated with cancer chemotherapy. Sixty patients were randomized into an experimental group (PMR), a placebo control group (relaxing music), and a true control group (no intervention). A statistically significant difference was found for trait anxiety scores across courses of chemotherapy within the different treatment groups; however, no statistical difference was found for state anxiety scores. This finding is perplexing in view of the theoretical constructs of state and trait anxiety and other research findings presented previously.

Frank[20] studied the effect of music therapy and guided visual imagery on anxiety associated with chemotherapy-induced nausea and vomiting. In a single group ($N = 15$), pretest- and posttest-designed study, musical tapes and visual imagery aided by a scenic poster were used beginning 15 minutes before chemotherapy and continuing through chemotherapy administration (2 hours). All subjects received antiemetic drugs before chemotherapy administration. State anxiety scores as measured by the STAI were reduced significantly ($p < .001$). In addition, a significant negative correlation was found between the length of time the subject listened to the music and the postchemotherapy state anxiety score ($r = -.4984$, $p < .05$).[19]

In summary, a variety of behavioral interventions have been used successfully to alleviate anxiety associated with a cancer diagnosis and treatment. Each intervention represents an independent nursing action to modify the anxiety response exhibited among persons with cancer.

Future Directions for Nursing Research

Anxiety has been reported to be present subjectively and objectively among patients diagnosed with cancer across the disease trajectory. The vague, uneasy feelings defined as anxiety may serve a protective or disabling function for the patient with cancer. However, assessment criteria used in collaboration with the perceptions of the patient to determine the individual level of anxiety at which interventions to reduce anxiety should be instituted lack reliability and validity.

Although beginning research efforts have focused on the effectiveness of a variety of independent nursing interventions in reducing anxiety among persons with cancer, studies have been limited by sample size and heterogeneity, cross-sectional designs, single measures of anxiety, use of anxiety as both an independent and a dependent variable, and lack of randomized control groups. Intervention studies for anxiety reduction among persons with cancer have concentrated on applying the intervention across cancer populations at a variety of points in the cancer trajectory, yet definition of criteria by which to select a specific intervention for a specific person may be impossible or, at best, subjective. Finally, the effect of anxiety reduction on patient outcomes such as information processing, physiologic responses to cancer and cancer therapy, psychosocial adaptation, and sense of control have not been corroborated.

DEPRESSION

Depression is a ubiquitous response to actual or potential loss. Since cancer represents a potential loss of not only life, but also body parts and functions, roles, and relationships, depression has been identified as one of the most common responses to cancer. Yet the differential diagnosis of depression among persons with cancer is complicated by the coexistence of signs and symptoms of disease and treatment that are similar to those of depression.[21] In addition, depression resulting from a predisposition within the personality must be differentiated from a depressed mood associated with an adjustment disorder as a result of changes caused by cancer.[22]

In either case, depression can influence the quality of life of persons with cancer and their significant others. However, empirical and clinical reports indicate that depression is an underdiagnosed response among persons with cancer and, probably more critical, undertreated.[23] In the following section, depression is defined, research on depression among persons with cancer is described, assessment criteria are discussed, and nursing interventions are outlined.

Operational Definition

The following operational definition of depression is presented:

- An individual exists with the ability to respond cognitively, behaviorally, and affectively to stimuli in the environment.

- The individual perceives certain goals for the future and attributes the possibilities for success to the self.

- The attempts of the individual to attain goals are blocked.

- The individual attributes the failure to attain goals to personal inadequacies.

- *The perceived loss of self-esteem results in a cluster of affective (worthlessness, hopelessness, guilt, sadness), behavioral (change in appetite, sleep disturbances, lack of energy, withdrawal, dependency), and cognitive (decreased ability to concentrate, indecisiveness, or suicidal ideation) responses defined as depression.*

Measurement Instruments

A variety of instruments is available to assess depression. The majority of these instruments were developed to assess depression in psychiatrically ill patients. Items cluster about the characteristics associated with major depression as described in the *Diagnostic and Statistical Manual of Mental Disorders-Revised* (DSM-III-R). Limited reliability and validity data with respect to use in oncology populations have been reported.

Hamilton Rating Scale for Depression

The Hamilton Rating Scale for Depression (HRS-D)[24] is a 17-item, self-report scale used to assess cognitive, behavioral, and physiologic signs and symptoms typical of depression. Each item is rated for severity from 0 to 2 or from 0 to 4. Scores on each item are summed to produce a total depression score. A total score of greater than 25 indicates severe depression; 18 to 24, moderate depression; 7 to 17, mild depression; and less than 6, no depression. Reliability and validity estimates for the instrument for nononcology populations include interrater reliability ($r = .90$); construct validity by factor analysis resulting in four factors (retarded depression, somatic symptoms, anxiety reaction, and insomnia).[24]

Beck Depression Inventory

The Beck Depression Inventory (BDI)[25] is a 21-item self-report scale used to assess symptoms of depression. Each item is composed of a set of statements, graduating in severity of symptoms, measured on a scale of 0 to 3, with a higher score representing a more severe symptom. The subject chooses the statement in the set that most closely describes his or her current feeling. Total scores for the BDI are based on the number and severity of symptoms experienced. Subjects scoring in the 0 to 4 range are classified as not or minimally depressed; in the 4 to 7 range, as mildly depressed; in the 8 to 15 range, as moderately depressed; and in the 16 to 42 range, as severely depressed. Reliability estimates among psychiatric populations include internal consistency (KR_{20} alpha coefficients ranging from .88 to .94).

Other instruments

In addition to the instruments presented, other personality and mood inventories with depression subscales have been used to quantify the level of depression. The Minnesota Multiphasic Personality Inventory (MMPI),[26] Psychosocial Adjustment to Illness Scale (PAIS),[27] and Profile of Mood States (POMS)[28] have been used most frequently in studies of depression among persons with cancer. Reliability and validity estimates for the total instrument as well as subscales are reported in administration and scoring manuals for each instrument.

Patterns of Occurrence

The occurrence of depression among persons with cancer has been described in the literature. Petty and Noyes[29] reported that moderate to severe depression was found in 17% to 25% of hospitalized cancer patients. At least 20% of adult cancer patients will have a clinically significant syndrome of depression during the course of the disease.[30-32]

Factors that affect the occurrence of depression among persons with cancer have been described. Andersen and Hacker[33] reported on the psychosexual adjustment of 15 patients treated surgically for vulvar cancer. Data were collected through a semistructured interview and battery of psychosocial questionnaires: Katz Social Adjustment Scale, Symptom Checklist-90, and Dyadic Adjustment Scale. A mean score of 12.3 on the BDI was obtained for the sample, indicating a mild to moderate level of depression among these patients. Activity scores were correlated significantly and negatively with the measures of psychologic distress.

Goldberg et al[34] reported on the relationship of the social environment and patient physical status to depression in 20 patients with lung cancer and their 18 spouses. Data were generated through a semistructured interview and a battery of psychological tests administered within 6 weeks of diagnosis and at 2-month intervals for 4 months. Physical status of the patient, as measured by the Karnofsky Scale, was related negatively to depressive symptoms as measured by POMS-D in patients.

The effects of age and marital status on emotional distress after mastectomy were studied by Metzger et al.[35] Data from interviews of 652 women who underwent a mastectomy 1 year before the study indicated that younger women were more likely to worry about disfigurement resulting from surgery but to have resources as buffers against depression. Married subjects were significantly less likely to worry about recurrence and experienced less depression.

Researchers have also attempted to differentiate depression associated with cancer from depression associated with a personality disorder. Robinson et al[36] conducted a study to determine if the degree of self-reported anxiety and depression that is attributed to having cancer differs from current or past history of anxiety and depression attributed to other life events in 57 patients presently being treated for cancer. Findings indicated that patients who reported a history of anxiety or depression for reasons other than cancer had significantly higher anxiety and depression scores than those who did not report preexisting anxiety or depression. Patients who reported a history of depression or anxiety due to the diagnosis of cancer had self-rating scores on anxiety and depression that did not differ significantly from those of patients who reported no problems or "normal" symptoms.

Evaluations for depression among 62 patients with a diagnosis of cancer were reported by Bukberg et al.[37] DSM-III-R criteria for major depressive episodes were used to evaluate the presence of depression.[38] Twenty-six patients (42%) met the criteria for major depression, 14% had depressive symptoms that did not meet the criteria for major depression, and 44% had no depressive affect. The factor most clearly associated with depression was physical performance as measured by the Karnofsky Scale. Qualitative differences between depression in psychiatric and cancer patients were found. No subjects were found to have psychotic depressive symptoms, melancholia, feelings of worthlessness, or suicidal ideation.

In addition to describing the occurrence of depression

among persons with cancer, researchers have studied the variations in occurrence and severity of depression across the disease trajectory. Layne et al[39] reported significant differences in levels of depression as measured by the MMPI-D among patients with a diagnosis of cancer in the terminal phase, patients with a diagnosis of cancer who had been told that they would survive for at least 5 years, family members of patients in the cancer groups, and a normal group. Depression scores for the terminal group were significantly greater than those of the family member and normal groups ($p < .05$). The nonterminal patient group also had depression scores greater than those of the family member and normal groups, although the differences were not statistically significant.

Depression also has been explored as a predictor of adjustment to a diagnosis of cancer. Morris et al[40] used standardized tests and structured interviews to identify factors that predicted psychological and social adjustment to mastectomy 2 years after surgery. High preoperative depression scores (HRS-D) were predictive of poor adjustment after mastectomy. Subjects who scored more than 10 on the HRS-D, with or without a history of depression, were significantly more likely to remain stressed by the mastectomy at 2 years ($p > .05$).

In summary, the focus of research related to depression among persons with cancer has been descriptive. The lack of assessment of preexisting depressive symptoms before the diagnosis of cancer, the presence of confounding physical and psychosocial responses related to the disease and treatment, and minimal reliability and validity estimates for instruments used among cancer populations result in significant limitations in previous research. Moreover, an emphasis on empirical studies that focus on independent nursing interventions to modify the depressive symptoms associated with the diagnosis of cancer is needed. With statistical modeling, knowledge of depressive responses within the context of other psychosocial variables inherent in the cancer experience may be enhanced.

Assessment Criteria

Reactive depression (situational) is defined as "an acute decrease in self-esteem or worth related to a threat to self competency" (p. 210).[15] Defining characteristics as established by NANDA are presented in Table 17-3.[15] Critical to establishing the diagnosis in physically ill persons is evaluation of selected defining characteristics commonly attributed to depression among the psychiatrically ill. Physiologic characteristics such as appetite disturbances, change in weight, sleep disturbance, and decreased energy are experienced frequently among persons with cancer as a result of disease or treatment. Furthermore, the psychosocial characteristics described for depression may occur in the person with cancer as a result of disease, treatment, or side effects (inability to concentrate, irritability, dependency, and anger). Therefore, the primary criteria for assessment of depression are that the characteristics are a change from previous functioning, are persistent,

TABLE 17-3 Defining Characteristics of Situational Depression

Expressions of hopelessness, despair
Inability to concentrate on reading, writing, conversation
Change in physical activities, eating, sleeping, sexual activity
Continual questioning of self-worth (self-esteem)
Feelings of failure (real or imagined)
Withdrawal from others to avoid possible rejection (real or imagined)
Threats or attempts to commit suicide
Suspicion and sensitivity to words and actions of others related to general lack of trust of others
Misdirected anger toward self
General irritability
Guilt feelings
Extreme dependency on others with related feelings of helplessness and anger

Source: Gordon M: Manual of Nursing Diagnosis. New York, McGraw-Hill, 1987.

occur for most of the day, occur more days than not, and are present for at least 2 weeks (p. 219).[38]

Nursing Interventions

The selection of nursing interventions for the treatment of patients with depression is based on identification of stimuli that have resulted in a loss of self-esteem as well as the defining characteristics present for the particular patient. If the patient presents with a long-standing history of depression, referral to another member of the health care team may be appropriate. Otherwise, concentration on the psychological and behavioral responses associated with depression offer beginning cues for selection of nursing interventions.

The nurse may begin by helping the patient to acknowledge feelings of hopelessness, despair, failure, anger, or guilt and by giving permission to discuss those feelings. Because the expression of the feelings is associated with a degree of risk-taking for the patient, the nurse must be open and accepting of the feelings. Acceptance is demonstrated by attentive listening, acknowledgment of the feelings, and exploration of methods to deal positively with the feelings.

Sensitivity to potential increased vulnerability of the patient who shares feelings is a necessity. The nurse must assume the responsibility for emotional exposure of the patient and plan systematically for professional follow-up. Expression of depressive feelings may be both time-consuming and overwhelming for the patient and nurse; consultation with other health care personnel, namely, clinical nurse specialists in psychiatry, psychologists, and psychiatrists, may be indicated.

Besides giving permission for expression of feelings, the nurse has the opportunity to assist the patient to reappraise the situation cognitively with respect to aspects of the cancer experience and perceptions of self-esteem and self-competency. Accurate information about the plan of care and personal responses to treatment form the basis of cognitive reappraisal of the situation. Helping the patient focus on immediate goals of care often reduces the overwhelming feelings of powerlessness and helplessness associated with a chronic, life-threatening illness. Focusing on positive abilities of the patient, contracting short-term goals of care that the patient can achieve, and reinforcing patient attempts and successes to meet established goals provide the framework for effective nursing interventions in caring for the patient with depression.

In the milieu of the cancer experience, physical symptoms of the disease and treatment as well as lack of motivation accompanying depression may limit the ability of the patient to meet basic needs. Significant others as well as health care professionals may perceive the patient as generally helpless even in areas in which the patient is able to function independently. Enhancing self-competency and self-esteem may be accomplished by providing information about and role modeling self-care behaviors, negotiating goals for increasing independence in self-care as well as decision making, facilitating social interaction with others, and encouraging physical mobility.

Future Directions for Nursing Research

Although most persons with cancer are able to cope with the demands of illness and treatment with minimal psychosocial distress, criteria by which to predict those patients for whom the demands exceed interpersonal and intrapersonal resources are ambiguous. Furthermore, criteria to establish the diagnosis among medically versus psychiatrically ill patients are unclear.

Nursing interventions designed to effect positive outcomes for the patient diagnosed with depression are inherently time-consuming and may represent an unacceptable cost-benefit ratio in the acute care setting in light of the physical care demanded. However, if the goal of oncology care includes the quality as well as quantity of life, then intervention studies to compare both the effectiveness as well as costs of care in both inpatient and community settings for patients with depression are warranted.

HOPELESSNESS

Hopelessness is often described in the literature as a response of patients to the cancer experience; however, the response appears not to pervade the experience of the cancer patient but rather waxes and wanes with changes in perceived health, relationships, and spirituality. Described as both a unique response as well as one of a cluster of characteristics seen in other responses, hopelessness has been studied primarily within the framework of psychiatrically ill patients. Recently, however, health care professionals in general and nurses in particular have demonstrated increased interest in hopelessness and hope as both independent and dependent variables influencing the quantity and quality of the cancer experience.

Operational Definition

Operationally, hopelessness can be defined as follows:

- An individual exists within time and space.

- The individual has thoughts, feelings, and behaviors in response to stimuli in the environment.

- The responses an individual has to stimuli are based on the significance of the stimuli, potential responses identified, and calculated probabilities of success in creating a desired future.

- The individual, as an aspect of humanity, recognizes significant areas of life for which limited or no alternatives are identified or the probabilities of success in creating a desired future approach zero—the perceived reality for the individual.

- In an attempt to protect the individual against the despair generated by these areas of life, the individual seeks a personal or spiritual relationship, anticipating that interactions will lead to understandable, meaningful, or constructive outcomes in the future.

- *The interaction of thoughts, feelings, and behaviors resulting from the inability to mobilize internal and external resources sufficient to achieve a probability of success greater than zero or to create an understandable, meaningful, or constructive outcome in the future is defined as hopelessness.*

Measurement Instruments
Beck Hopelessness Scale

The Beck Hopelessness Scale (BHS)[41] is a 20-item, true-false scale designed to measure hopelessness in psychiatrically ill patients. Scores are calculated by summing the scores on each statement. Scores range from 0 to 20, with a higher score representing a higher level of hopelessness. Scores of 0 to 3 represent no or minimal hopelessness; 4 to 8, mild hopelessness; 9 to 14, moderate hopelessness; and 15 to 20, severe hopelessness. Reliability estimates for the instrument include internal consistency as measured by the KR_{20} reliability coefficient = .93 among a sample of suicide attempters; concurrent validity between clinical ratings of hopelessness and instrument ratings ($r = .74$, $p < .001$); face validity established by a panel of psychiatric experts; and construct validity through factor analysis resulting in three factors (feelings about the future, loss of motivation, and future expectations)[41] with Eigenvalues > 1.000.

Nowotny Hope Scale

Conceptualized as a polar opposite to hopelessness, hopefulness has been measured by a number of instruments developed by nurse researchers. The Nowotny Hope Scale (NHS)[42] is a 29-item scale designed to measure hope on six dimensions: confidence in outcomes, relates to others, possibility of a future, spiritual beliefs, active involvement, and comes from within.[42] For each of the positively and negatively worded statements, the subject is asked to respond on a 4-point, Likert-type scale (1 = strongly agree to 4 = strongly disagree). Reliability and validity estimates for the instrument include internal consistency as calculated by Cronbach's coefficient alpha = 0.90; item-total correlations ranging from 0.3 to 0.7; item to subscale correlations ranging from 0.4 to 0.8; concurrent validity with the BHS ($r = .47, p = .001$); and construct validity through factor analysis resulting in six factors with Eigenvalues ranging from 9.8 to 1.4.[42]

Herth Hope Scale

The Herth Hope Scale (HHS)[43] is a 32-item self-report scale to which subjects respond either "applies to me" or "does not apply to me" to each item. Responses on each item are summed to produce a total hope score ranging from 0 to 32, with a higher score representing higher levels of hope. Reliability and validity estimates among persons with cancer include internal consistency as determined by Cronbach's coefficient alpha = 0.89; and construct validity through factor analysis resulting in three factors—positive expectancies, sense of personal competency and mutuality, and temporality with future orientation.[43]

Patterns of Occurrence

In recent years, the interest of health care professionals in the relationship of hope and hopelessness to the cancer experience has resulted in numerous anecdotal articles, a few descriptive studies, and a limited number of intervention studies. As early as 1966, Schmale and Iker[44] conducted a study of 40 women with abnormal cervical cytology suspicious of cancer. To test the hypothesis that the experience of specific feelings may facilitate or permit the clinical appearance of disease,[44] the researchers conducted an interview and administered a battery of psychological tests the day after a cone biopsy was done under general anesthesia. Content analysis of interviews was compared with preestablished criteria for hopelessness potential. A determination of "cancer" or "no cancer" was made for each subject. Thirty-one subjects (77.5%) were assigned to the correct grouping (x_c^2, 7.343; df, 1; $p = .007$).

Subsequent studies of hope among persons with cancer were focused on concept clarification, describing levels of hope across the disease trajectory, or instrument development for measuring hope. Using a grounded theory

TABLE 17-4 Induced Dimensions of Hopefulness Among Adolescents

Dimension	Definition
Forced effort	The degree to which an adolescent tries to take on artificially a more positive view
Personal possibilities	The extent to which an adolescent believes that second chances for the self may exist
Expectations of a better tomorrow	The degree to which an adolescent has a positive although nonspecific future orientation
Anticipation of a personal future	The extent to which an adolescent identifies specific and positive future possibilities for self

Source: Hinds PS: Adolescent hopefulness in illness and health. Adv Nurs Sci 10:79-88, 1988.

methodology, Hinds[45] developed an empirically derived definition of hopefulness through interviews with healthy adolescents, inpatient adolescents on a substance abuse unit, and a diagnostically heterogeneous adolescent group with cancer.

The induced definition of hopefulness had four dimensions that emerged from the data from the healthy and substance abuse adolescents (Table 17-4).[45] An additional attribute emerged from the adolescent cancer group, "the concern for and a focus on others in addition to self" (p. 85).[45] Thus, the resulting definition became "the degree to which an adolescent possesses a comforting or life-sustaining, reality-based belief that a positive future exists for self or others."[45] These data form the basis for additional study of the concept among adults.

In a similar study, the phenomena of hope and the hoping process were examined among 35 elderly patients with a diagnosis of cancer.[46] Hope was defined as a multidimensional dynamic life force characterized by confident yet uncertain anticipation of realistically possible and personally significant desirable future good having implications for action and for interpersonal relatedness (p. 380).[46] Two spheres of hope, generalized and particularized, were identified, and six dimensions of hope were described—affective, cognitive, behavioral, affiliative, temporal, and contextual.

In a report on the development of an instrument to measure hope after a stressful event, Nowotny[42] described levels of hope among a sample of 150 patients with cancer. Scores on the NHS for the cancer patient group were not significantly different from scores of a sample of 156 well adults. Data were not collected on type of diagnosis, length of time since diagnosis, or type of treatment for the cancer patient sample.

Zook and Yasko[47] found hope levels decreased as time since diagnosis increased among a group of 26 patients with cancer receiving chemotherapy. In contrast, Greene et al[48] reported no correlation between hope level and length of time since diagnosis.

The focus of more recent studies has been the description of the relationship of hope to other psychosocial variables in the cancer experience. Herth[43] reported a descriptive study to investigate the relationship between hope and coping in 120 adult patients with cancer undergoing chemotherapy in a variety of care settings. A significant relationship was found between level of hope and level of coping among subjects in hospital, outpatients, and home settings ($p < .05$). In addition, strength of religious convictions and performance of family role responsibilities, measured on one-item scales, were significantly related to the variables of hope and coping regardless of setting: subjects with a strong religious faith had significantly higher mean scores on the HHS than subjects with weak, unsure, or lost faith or who were without faith. Subjects who reported little or no interference in performing family role responsibilities had a significantly ($p < .05$) higher mean score on the HHS than did the group indicating severe interference.

Raleigh[49] studied 45 patients with cancer and 45 individuals with a nonthreatening chronic illness to describe the relationship between hope, locus of control, factors of illness, and personal factors. Raleigh reported no significant relationship between the level of hope and the identified personal and illness factors, yet these findings have been challenged.

To examine the relationship between hopelessness and locus of control, helpfulness of religious beliefs, and support from family and friends, Brandt[50] studied a sample of 31 women with breast cancer. Although all patients were receiving their first course of chemotherapy, variability existed in the time elapsed since initial diagnosis; that is, 42% of the sample had been diagnosed less than 6 months, while 26% of the sample had been diagnosed more than 24 months. Results indicate that the mean hopelessness score as measured by the BHS was 2.48, indicating minimal hopelessness. A statistically significant correlation ($r = .37$, $p < .05$) was found between hopelessness scores and locus of control scores (as measured by the Rotter I-E Locus of Control Scale). Patients who exhibited a more external locus of control expressed a greater level of hopelessness.[50] Perceived helpfulness of religious beliefs in coping with illness as measured by a one-item scale was found to be correlated significantly ($r = -.32$, $p < .05$) with lower levels of hopelessness. The author indicated minimal variability of scores on the religious beliefs question. Support from family and friends as measured by a one-item scale did not produce sufficient variability in scores to allow a Pearson correlation coefficient to be calculated.

Stoner[51] studied the relationship between personal and situational factors and hope in 58 white adults with cancer. Higher levels of hope ($p = .10$) were associated with being female, receipt of adequate information about disease and treatments, adherence by the subjects to their religious belief systems throughout illness, and lower socioeconomic status. Inability to carry out family role responsibilities, adverse effects of treatment, protracted illness, and greater severity of illness were not found to be associated with lower levels of hope.

In a subsequent study, Stoner and Keampfer[52] examined the effect of information with respect to life expectancy and phase of illness on levels of hope among a heterogeneous sample of 55 cancer patients. Although data indicated no significant differences in levels of hope between subjects according to the phase of illness (no evidence of disease, ongoing treatment, or terminal stage), a significant main effect for recalled life expectancy information on hope was shown ($F = 4.21$, $p < .05$). Subjects who did not remember receiving information about life expectancy had higher levels of hope than subjects who remembered receiving information.[52]

The relationship between hopefulness and participation styles with respect to treatment was studied among a sample of 256 patients with a diagnosis of cancer.[53] Selected findings of Stoner[52] were supported. The mean score on the BHS for the sample was 2.8, indicating minimal hopelessness. Levels of hope were found to correlate positively with medical status ($p < .05$); preference for active involvement in self-care ($p < .05$); and desire for as much information as possible ($p < .001$).

Hope as an intervening variable has been studied.[54] The relationship between locus of control, hope, and disease-free interval was examined among a convenience sample of 34 postmenopausal women with stage II breast cancer. Internal health locus of control was not found to be correlated significantly with disease-free interval; however, hope was found to be correlated positively and significantly ($p < .05$) with disease-free interval. Moreover, stressful life events were found to be intervening variables that had a significant negative correlation with disease-free interval.

Thus, hopefulness and hopelessness have been implicated in the development of cancer and in the quantity and quality of life after diagnosis of cancer. However, consistent conceptualization of hope and hopelessness remains elusive in the empirical studies reported. Ideally, future efforts in determining the relationship of hope and cancer will be targeted to demonstrate the biophysical-psychosocial connection between the variables.

Assessment Criteria

Hopelessness has been characterized by cognitive, affective, and behavioral responses (Table 17-5).[15] Few studies, however, have been conducted to establish the reliability and validity of the defining characteristics among clinical populations. Of even greater concern is the ability of the clinician to differentiate hopelessness from similar concepts such as depression and powerlessness using the accepted defining characteristics.

TABLE 17-5 Nursing Diagnosis: Hopelessness

Definition	A subjective state in which an individual sees limited or no alternative or personal choices available and is unable to mobilize energy on own behalf
Defining characteristics	Passivity Decreased verbalization Decreased affect Verbalization of despondent or hopeless content Lack of initiative Decreased response to stimuli Lack of involvement in care Turning away from speaker Closing eyes Shrugging in response to speaker Decreased appetite Increased sleep

Source: Gordon M: Manual of Nursing Diagnosis. New York, McGraw-Hill, 1987.

Nursing Interventions

Interventions for decreasing hopelessness and fostering hope among persons with cancer have been derived before development of conceptual and theoretical formulations. Based on conceptual models of the nature of hope and related variables, the following categories of interventions have been suggested: enhancing reality surveillance, fostering supportive relationships, enhancing personal power and abilities, and creating a future perspective.[55,56] Specific suggestions for implementation of each category are presented in Table 17-6.[55,56]

Future Directions for Nursing Research

Hope has been identified as a critical component of cancer care. As such, the necessity of conceptualizing hope and hopelessness within the context of the cancer experience, validating the defining characteristics of hope and hopelessness, describing the association of hope and hopelessness to other psychosocial variables, and evaluating the effectiveness of specific nursing interventions in fostering hope or protecting against hopelessness is apparent.

ALTERED SEXUAL HEALTH

The diagnosis of cancer poses potential threats to sexuality, how one perceives the self, how one perceives how others see the self, and how one behaves as a sexual being. As the nature of cancer has changed from an acute to a chronic illness, concerns of health care providers have

TABLE 17-6 Interventions to Foster Hopefulness

Category	Interventions
Assist with reality surveillance	Review changes in and current health status Seek perceptions of patient with respect to health Confirm accurate perception Correct misconceptions of reality Encourage discussion of reality with others in same situation
Reinforce personal power and ability	Review perceived strengths of patient and family Include patient in planning care, goals, schedules Encourage review of past successes in stressful times Reward approximations of goals Encourage value of use of needed external resources
Encourage supportive relationships	Review number, types, and availability of supportive relationships Assist in helping patient ask for support needed Encourage continued contacts with supportive persons Respect relationship of patient to higher being Encourage expression of faith, if applicable
Create a future perspective	Review past occasions for hope Discuss meaning of hope from patient perspective Establish short-term goals with patient and family Evaluate progress in achieving goals on routine basis Encourage expressions of hopes for future

Sources: Clark JC: Hope as a critical factor in the cancer experience, in Pritchard AP (ed): Cancer Nursing: A Revolution in Care, Proceeding of the Fifth International Conference on Cancer Nursing. London, Macmillan, 1989, pp 117-119. Dufault K, Martocchio BC; Hope: Its spheres and dimensions. Nurs Clin North Am 20:379-391, 1985.

expanded beyond survival to include factors that affect the quality of survival. Sexual health is one such factor.

Operational Definition

Operationally, sexuality can be defined as follows:

- An individual exists who has the ability to express himself or herself physically, psychologically, and socially with other human beings.

- The ability of the individual to distinguish self from and express self with others based on anatomic, physiologic, developmental, and psychosocial factors is defined as sexuality.

- The satisfactory, consistent, and rewarding expression of and distinction by one's sexuality results in a state of sexual health for the individual.

- The individual perceives a stimulus that impairs distinction or expression of sexuality.

- *The inability to express one's sexuality consistent with personal needs and preferences is defined as altered sexual health.*

Measurement Instruments
Derogatis Sexual Functioning Inventory

The Derogatis Sexual Functioning Inventory (DSFI)[57] is a 245-item, self-report instrument designed to measure the multidimensional concept of sexuality. Reported reliability and validity estimates include test-retest reliabilities for 10 subscales ranging from 0.42 to 0.96; internal consistency coefficients ranging from 0.56 to 0.97; and construct validity through factor analysis that revealed seven factors (body image, psychologic distress, heterosexual drive, autoeroticism, gender role, sexual satisfaction, and sexual precociousness).[57]

Sexual Adjustment Questionnaire

The Sexual Adjustment Questionnaire (SAQ)[58] is a 108-item instrument designed to measure sexual adjustment over time among patients with head and neck cancers. The questionnaire is completed by the subject at three separate points in time: Section A (37 items), 4 to 6 weeks after treatment; Section B (30 items), retrospective assessment before the diagnosis of cancer; and Section C (39 items), 16 to 20 weeks after treatment. Items include some questions evaluated on a 5-point Likert scale, several open-ended questions, and questions that require an explanation from the subject. Each section is composed of 7 subsections: desire, relationship, activity arousal, orgasm, techniques, and satisfaction. Scores on each item are summed to produce a total score for the subsection. High scores indicate more positive feelings of functioning, greater variety of sexual methods and activities, or a long-term relationship with a single partner. Reliability and validity estimates for the instrument include: test-retest reliability (2 to 4 weeks and 10 to 12 weeks apart) with Pearson correlation coefficients for the subsections ranging from .5389 to .9374; content validity evaluation by a panel of experts; and construct validity established by known-group technique (healthy subjects would be expected to score higher than cancer patients).

Patterns of Occurrence

The sequelae associated with radical surgery, radiation, chemotherapy, and biotherapy may threaten the sexual health of persons with cancer. Early studies on the effects of cancer on sexual health focused on barriers to return to previous levels of sexual function or, more specifically, intercourse. Anecdotal reports and descriptive studies provided the basis for identifying the potential risks to sexual health for site-specific and treatment-specific patient populations. Recently, however, researchers have expanded the concept of sexual health and sexuality to include the issues of self-concept and perceptions and behaviors of significant others.

Sexual behaviors

Abitbol and Davenport[59] published data related to the impact of treatment for cervical cancer on sexual function. Subjects (28 treated with radiation therapy only, 32 treated with surgery, and 15 treated with a combination of surgery and radiation) were interviewed about their sexual life before disease, sexual life 1 year after treatment, and other changes in sexual functioning. Approximately 40% of patients ($N = 75$) reported a decrease or abstinence in sexual activity after treatment. The radiotherapy group had the highest percentage of subjects reporting a decrease in sexual activity (25%). Other changes in sexual functioning identified primarily by the radiotherapy group were lack of libido (43%), pain or discomfort with intercourse (39%), shortened or narrowed vagina (54%), and fear of recurrence (15%). The authors recommended that clinicians assume a proactive posture in addressing the sexual concerns of cancer patients treated with radiation therapy regardless of age.

Subsequently, Jenkins[60] discussed the self-reported sexual changes in 27 women treated for endometrial and cervical cancer with surgery and radiation therapy. A statistically significant ($p < .05$) negative change in the frequency of intercourse, frequency of desire, frequency of orgasm, and enjoyment of intercourse was reported after treatment. Additional significant findings of the study included that 59% of the sample had received no preparation or information about sexual functioning, the majority of sexual information given was verbal versus written, and nurses had not provided any of the information about sexual functioning.

These findings were supported in a study of 60 women newly diagnosed with gynecologic cancers.[61] Twenty-nine of the subjects were sexually active before diagnosis. However, none of these subjects continued to have sexual intercourse after diagnosis either on recommendation of the physician or fear that intercourse would increase the risk for vaginal bleeding or discharge.

Surgery also has been implicated in changes in sexual health among women with vulvar cancer. Andersen and Hacker[62] reported on the psychosexual adjustment of 15 patients treated surgically for vulvar cancer. Data were collected through a semistructured interview and battery of psychosocial questionnaires. Measures of sexual functioning indicated that the sample reported limited capacity for sexual arousal, considerable sexual anxiety, inadequate sexual relationships, a discrepancy between actual and ideal frequency of intercourse, and lower body image scores than reported for healthy women.

The sexual function and psychosocial reactions among 25 women who had undergone vulvectomy and 15 of their partners indicated that more than two thirds of the patients reported a decrease in frequency of intercourse from pretreatment levels.[63] Ten women ceased sexual intercourse completely. Half the women reported being dissatisfied with sexual relationships and the occurrence of low spirits, lack of respect for their body, and not feeling like a "proper woman." These data are consistent with the findings of Jenkins[60] in that between 25% and 33% of patients perceived the information given to them before treatment as inadequate.

However, findings from related studies among women with breast cancer have not been consistent with the changes reported among women with gynecologic cancers. Woods and Earp[64] reported on 49 patients cured of stage I and II breast cancer. Four years after therapy, 81% of the sample reported no differences in sexual frequency and 63% reported being satisfied with sexual relationships. These findings were supported by the work of Jamison et al[65] who interviewed 41 women with breast cancer. Seventy-six percent of the sample reported that the mastectomy had resulted in no difference or a positive effect on sexual satisfaction or orgasmic ability. Only 2.7% reported a decrease in sexual activity or interest.

In contrast, Taylor et al[66] reported changes in the levels of affectionate behavior in the marriage ($r = .51$, $p < .001$) and patient perception of frequency of intercourse ($r = .32$, $p < .03$) that were associated with poor psychosocial adjustment among 78 women diagnosed and treated for breast cancer. Patients treated with modified radical mastectomy had significantly higher concern about body disfigurement and were affected significantly more negatively with respect to marital affection and sexual intercourse levels than were patients treated with lumpectomy.

Thus, data indicate that women with gynecologic cancers in general and those treated with radiation therapy are at risk for changes in sexual activity. In contrast, the diagnosis of breast cancer and treatment with surgery do not appear to place the patient at increased risk for changes in the frequency of sexual intercourse but, rather, for changes in self-concept.

Although empirical data are available for evaluating the potential risks of cancer and treatment among females, such data for males are limited. Blackmore[67] reported on the impact of orchidectomy on the sexuality of men with testicular cancer. Self-report questionnaires were distributed to three groups of subjects: group I, 20 men with stage I germ cell testicular tumors treated with unilateral orchidectomy within 2 years before the study; group II, 10 men who had undergone unilateral orchidectomy within 2 years before the study for reasons other than

cancer; and group III, 15 men who had no history of cancer or testicular problems. Five sections of the DSFI (sexual drive, symptoms, affect, body image, and sexual satisfaction) were used as the basis for data collection. No statistically significant differences were found on any outcome sexuality variables among the three groups. In contrast, Schover et al[68] found significant sexual morbidity among a sample of 84 men with a diagnosis of seminoma who were treated with radiation therapy. Problems reported included reduced semen volume (49%), reduced intensity of orgasm (33%), low rates of sexual activity (19%), low sexual desire (12%), erectile dysfunction (15%), difficulty reaching orgasm (10%), and premature ejaculation (14%).

Although treatment of prostatic cancer can affect sexual functioning (impotence and reduced frequency of intercourse and orgasm), limited empirical data are available to quantify the occurrence of sexual changes.[69] Banker[70] studied the preservation of potency among 100 men with prostate cancer treated with external radiation therapy. Subjects were interviewed before radiation therapy and again 1 year after treatment concerning frequency of intercourse, changes in sexual activity levels over the past 1 to 3 years, and ability to achieve and maintain a full erection. Forty-three percent of subjects ($n = 10$) who reported having intercourse with full erections less than three times per month before therapy maintained potency after treatment, compared with 73% of subjects ($n = 19$) who had intercourse with full erection more than three times per month.

In summary, researchers have identified the potential assaults to sexual health among males with genitourinary cancers, yet the data are limited with respect to threats to sexual health among persons with cancers of the head and neck, lung, and gastrointestinal tract. Also of interest is the lack of research related to the perceptions of significant others with respect to sexuality and perceptions of the patient with respect to self-concept.

Self-concept

Self-concept is defined as the total self-appraisal of appearance, background and origins, abilities, resources, attitudes, and feelings that culminate as a directing force in behavior.[71] Newman et al[72] reported on the effect of Hickman catheters on the self-esteem of patients with leukemia. Self-esteem was measured on admission, on day 5, and on day 30.[73] Consecutive patients admitted with acute nonlymphocytic leukemia (ANLL) were assigned to two groups based on adequacy of venous access. Thirty patients were assigned to each group. Patients who received a Hickman catheter had initial self-esteem scores similar to and even slightly higher than those who did not. Self-esteem in both groups remained similar over the 30-day study period. However, one may question the appropriateness of the use of the Purpose in Life test to measure the self-esteem concept.

In contrast to the minimal surgical incision involved with a Hickman catheter placement, Weddington et al[74] studied the psychological outcome of extremity sarcoma survivors undergoing amputation ($n = 14$) or limb salvage procedures ($n = 19$). No significant differences between group scores of cognitive capacity, symptoms, mood, body image changes, physical function, adjustment to illness and surgery, and lifetime prevalence of psychiatric disorders before or after surgery were noted.

Alopecia is one of the most common physiologic responses to chemotherapy. Baxley et al[75] studied the effect of alopecia on the body image of 40 patients with cancer receiving chemotherapy. Subjects were divided into two groups based on the presence of alopecia. Each subject completed the Body-Cathexis-Self-Cathexis (BC-SC) Scale.[76] Significant differences on body cathexis scores ($t = 4.34$, $p < .001$) and self-cathexis scores ($t = 4.04$, $p < .0001$) were found between patients with and without alopecia. In addition, comparisons of scores for female and male patients in the alopecia group indicated a significant difference ($t = 2.91$, $p < .0009$) in that men with alopecia scored higher, indicating that they had a lower self-image than women with alopecia.

Evaluation of the impact of radical versus conservative surgery on disease-related and adjustment-related outcomes has been studied. Kemeny et al[77] conducted a study of the differences in the psychosocial effects of mastectomy ($n = 27$) versus segmentectomy ($n = 25$) in women who were entered in a prospective randomized protocol for treatment of primary breast cancer. Questionnaires that were designed to evaluate psychosocial responses to treatment were sent to each subject who was at least 6 months past completion of treatment. Seven items were used to evaluate the emotional reaction to body image. Although responses to the items clustered around 3.0, "not sure," for the mastectomy patients, the segmentectomy patients had a significantly more positive assessment of themselves. Patients were asked to evaluate retrospectively changes in physical attractiveness before surgery, 6 months after surgery, and 6 months after completion of

therapy. The mastectomy group rated themselves as significantly less physically attractive at 6 months after surgery ($p < .003$) and at the time of the questionnaire ($p < .04$). Mastectomy patients also had a significantly lower rating of femininity 6 months after surgery ($p < .01$) than patients in the segmentectomy group.[77]

In summary, the majority of empirical studies on the impact of cancer on sexual health have been descriptive in design and focused primarily on the effects of cancer and treatment on the frequency of sexual behaviors, particularly intercourse and orgasm, or on self-concept among females with gynecologic and breast cancer or on males with testicular and prostate cancer. However, the issues of perception of significant others' responses to the physical and psychological sequelae of cancer remain understudied. Additional empirical data are needed on the interaction of other variables, such as age, depression, and activity status, on the physical as well as psychosocial aspects of sexual health.

Assessment Criteria

Two nursing diagnoses related to sexual health have been approved by NANDA—sexual dysfunction and altered sexuality patterns.[15] Defining characteristics for each diagnosis are presented in Table 17-7.[15] Differential diagnosis of the two responses based on defining characteristics is conceptually ambiguous in that the defining characteristic for altered sexuality patterns (reported difficulties, limitations, or changes in sexual behaviors or activities) provides the broad categories of the defining characteristics for sexual dysfunction.

Although conceptualization of the diagnoses related to sexual health requires clarification, the defining characteristics do emphasize subjective as well as objective criteria for evaluation of sexual health. Like other responses described in this chapter, the subjective responses and per-

TABLE 17-7 Nursing Diagnoses: Altered Sexual Health

Nursing Diagnosis	Definition	Defining Characteristics
Altered sexual patterns	The state in which an individual expresses concern regarding sexuality	Reported difficulties, limitations, or changes in sexual behaviors or activities
Sexual dysfunction	Perceived problem in achieving desired satisfaction of sexuality	Verbalizations of problem in sexuality Alterations in achieving perceived sex role Actual or perceived limitation imposed by disease or therapy Conflicts involving values Alteration in achieving sexual satisfaction Inability to achieve desired sexual satisfaction Frequent seeking of confirmation of desirability Alteration in relationship with significant other Change of interest in self and others

Source: Gordon M: Manual of Nursing Diagnosis. New York, McGraw-Hill, 1987.

TABLE 17-8   Levels of Sexual Counseling: The PLISSIT Model

P (Permission)	LI (Limited Information)	SS (Specific Suggestions)	IT (Intensive Therapy)
Legitimize sexual concerns	Anticipatory guidance with respect to sexual concerns	Cognitive reappraisal	Referral to professional therapist
Express sexual concerns with partner and health care team	Provide information needed for rehabilitation	Coping skills for changes experienced in communication, roles, relationships	
		Modify behaviors to accommodate limitations imposed by cancer or treatment	

Source: Adapted from Shipes E, Lehr S: Sexuality and the male cancer patient. Cancer Nurs 5:375-381, 1982.

ceptions of the individual and, in this case, significant others must be considered when identifying a problem and planning care.

Nursing Interventions

Interventions for alterations in sexual health are based on assessment of the subjective perceptions and objective responses of the patient and significant others and careful delineation of the etiology of the problem. From the review of the literature, one is able to identify the most common etiologies of alterations to sexual health related to a diagnosis of cancer and the primary categories of nursing interventions.[78-80] However, the specific approach, suggestions, and resources used to treat the problem must be guided by the etiology of the problem and the perceptions and motivations of the patient or significant other.

Annon[78] has described a simple hierarchy of interventions for sexual problems known as the PLISSIT model (Table 17-8).[80] The system implies that for many problems, the simple acknowledgement and discussion of the perception of change in sexual health may be sufficient to help the patient or significant other resolve the problem. For other problems, especially those that existed before the diagnosis of cancer, referral to a professional for intensive individual or couple therapy may be indicated. For a detailed discussion on this intervention, see Chapter 29, Altered Body Image and Sexuality.

Approaches to treatment of changes in sexual health identified in the literature include education and counseling, yet few empirical studies have addressed the effectiveness of such interventions in ameliorating the symptoms associated with altered sexual health. Capone et al[81] examined the effects of counseling on psychosocial rehabilitation in a study of 56 patients with gynecologic cancers and 41 patients who met the same criteria but served as controls. Forty-one (73%) of the experimental group and 25 (61%) of the control group were sexually active before initiation of treatment and not more than 6 weeks after diagnosis. Subjects in both groups were interviewed and completed a battery of psychological tests (Self-Rating Symptom Scale, Profile of Mood States, and Tennessee Self-Concept Scale). The experimental group received individual counseling based on crisis intervention principles. Counseling included helping the patient to shape reality-based expectations, facilitating adaptive changes in behaviors, enhancing reintegration of self, and teaching information-processing skills. Interviews and testing were repeated at 3, 6, and 12 months after treatment. Significant differences were found in comparative frequencies of intercourse between the counseling and control groups at 3 ($p < .04$), 6 ($p < .007$), and 12 ($p < .05$) months. Counseling was found to have a positive effect on the resumption of sexual intercourse during the first year after treatment.[81]

More recently, Cain et al[82] described the psychosocial benefits of a cancer support group for women with a diagnosis of gynecologic cancer. After a psychosocial assessment within 1 month of diagnosis, subjects were assigned to one of three counseling groups: standard mode ($n = 31$), thematic individual mode ($n = 21$), and thematic group ($n = 28$). Each intervention was conducted for 8 weeks. Postcounseling data at 2 weeks and 6 months were obtained. Before the intervention, many of the subjects had significant disruption in sexual relationships. Women in the thematic individual and group counseling categories described significantly better sexual relationships at 6 months compared with baseline data ($F = 4.10$, $p < .02$).[82]

The two studies described are examples of innovative approaches to modify the threat of cancer to sexual health. However, the outcomes by which the effectiveness of the interventions were measured focus primarily on resumption of sexual intercourse. One might question that if sexual health is determined by how individuals perceive themselves, how they perceive that others see them, and how they behave in relationships with others, why were significant others not included in the intervention?

A second concern with respect to the interventions described is the lack of screening of patients for participation. Resource consumption of personnel, time, physical facilities, and materials required by such programs must be weighed against the benefits of the program. Therefore, selection of high risk patients for sexual dysfunction to participate in the program may increase the likelihood that sexual morbidity would be reduced. Screening would increase the probability of identifying those patients and partners with preexisting problems that may require more intensive therapy. For more information on this subject, see Chapter 29.

Future Directions for Nursing Research

Although sexual health is important, health care professionals have assigned limited value to and assumed a limited perspective of sexual health in relation to cancer care. Increasingly complex, multimodal, and lengthy treatment for cancer increases the risks of changes in sexual health among people diagnosed with cancer and their significant others.

Development of clinical and research instruments that have established reliability and validity for assessment of sexual health dimensions among people with cancer are needed. In addition, multimethods of assessing sexual health not only in the patient but also from the perspective of significant others are required if the interrelationships of the complex factors that contribute to sexual health are to be understood.

Definition, labeling, and validation of changes in sexual health among persons with cancer that require professional intervention are mandated by the level of concept clarification that currently exists. In addition, the effectiveness of educational, counseling, and anticipatory guidance interventions for selected patient and significant other populations should be evaluated.

CONCLUSION

Cancer threatens both the quantity and quality of life for the person who is faced with complex treatment plans, the uncertainty of recurrence, and integration of changed concepts of self, roles, and relationships resulting from the disease and treatment. The responses discussed in this chapter represent high-incidence phenomena described in the literature. One can see how little professionals know and understand about the incidence, contributing factors, variations of response, and long-term consequences of responses for the individual experiencing cancer. Thus, interventions designed to minimize the dysfunctional effects of the experience of cancer are, by the nature of our understanding of the phenomena, limited to "shot-gun," trial-and-error efforts. The specificity of interventions to particular patients based on a systematic appraisal of intrapersonal, interpersonal, social, and economic resources awaits the future.

REFERENCES

1. Spielberger C, Gorsuch R, Lushene R: Manual for the state-trait anxiety inventory. Palo Alto, Calif, Consulting Psychologists Press, 1970.
2. Lucente FE, Fleck S: A study of hospitalization anxiety in 408 medical and surgical patients. Psychosom Med 34:304-312, 1972.
3. Gottesman D, Lewis MS: Differences in crisis reactions among cancer and surgery patients. J Consult Clin Psychol 50:381-388, 1982.
4. Scott DW: Anxiety, critical thinking, and information processing during and after breast biopsy. Nurs Res 32:24-28, 1983.
5. Morris J, Royle GT: Choice of surgery for early breast cancer: Pre- and postoperative levels of clinical anxiety and depression in patients and their husbands. Br J Surg 74:1017-1019, 1987.
6. Oberst MT, Scott DW: Post discharge distress in surgically treated cancer patients and their spouses. Res Nurs Health 11:223-233, 1988.
7. Gottschalk LA, Hoigaard-Martin J: The emotional impact of mastectomy. Psychiatr Res 17:153-167, 1986.
8. Irwin PH, Kramer S, Diamond NH, et al: Sex differences in psychological distress during definitive radiation therapy for cancer. J Psychosoc Oncol 4:63-75, 1986.
9. Andersen BL, Tewfik HH: Psychological reactions to radiation therapy: Reconsideration of the adaptive aspects of anxiety. J Personal Soc Psychol 48:1024-1032, 1985.
10. Andersen BL, Karlsson JA, Anderson B, et al: Anxiety and cancer treatment: Response to stressful radiotherapy. Health Psychol 3:535-551, 1984.
11. Redd WH, Andrykowski MA: Behavioral intervention in cancer treatment: Controlling aversion reactions to chemotherapy. J Consult Clin Psychol 50:1018-1029, 1982.
12. Cassileth BR, Lusk EJ, Walsh WP: Anxiety levels in patients with malignant disease. Hospice J 2:57-69, 1986.
13. Cella DF, Pratt A, Holland JC: Persistent anticipatory nausea, vomiting, and anxiety in cured Hodgkin's disease patients after completion of chemotherapy. Am J of Psychiatry 143:641-643, 1986.
14. Carey MP, Burish TG: Anxiety as a predictor of behavioral therapy outcome for cancer chemotherapy patients. J Consult Clin Psychol 53:860-865, 1985.
15. Gordon M: Manual of Nursing Diagnosis. New York, McGraw-Hill, 1987.
16. Scandrett S: Cognitive reappraisal, in Bulechek GM, McCloskey J (eds): Nursing Interventions: Treatments for Nursing Diagnosis. Philadelphia, WB Saunders, 1985, pp 49-57.
17. Miller JF: Coping with Chronic Illness: Overcoming Powerlessness. Philadelphia, FA Davis, 1983.
18. Johnson J: The effects of a patient education course on persons with a chronic illness. Cancer Nurs 5:117-123, 1982.
19. Cotanch PH, Strum S: Progressive muscle relaxation as antiemetic therapy for cancer patients. Oncol Nurs Forum 14:33-37, 1987.
20. Frank JM: The effects of music therapy and guided visual imagery on chemotherapy induced nausea and vomiting. Oncol Nurs Forum 12:47-52, 1985.
21. Davis T, Jensen L: Identifying depression in medical patients. Image: J Nurs Scholarship 20:191-95, 1988.
22. Robinson JK, Boshier ML, Dansak DA, et al: Depression and anxiety in cancer patients: Evidence for different causes. J Psychosom Res 29:133-138, 1985.

23. Neilson AC, Williams TA: Depression in ambulatory medical patients. Arch Gen Psychiatry 37:999-1004, 1980.

24. Hamilton M: A rating scale for depression. J Neurol Neurosurg Psychiatry 23:56-62, 1960.

25. Beck AT, Beamesderfer A: Assessment of depression: The depression inventory, in Pichot P, Olivier-Martin R (eds): Psychological Measurements in Psychopharmacology: Modern Problems in Pharmopsychiatry (Vol 7). Basel, Karger, 1974, pp 151-169.

26. Nelson LD: Measuring depression in a clinical population using the MMPI. J Consult Clin Psychol 55:788-790, 1987.

27. Derogatis LR, Melisaratos N: The DSFI: A multidimensional measure of sexual functioning. J Sex Marital Therapy 5:244-281, 1979.

28. McNair DM, Lorr M, Droppleman LF: Profile of mood states. San Diego, Calif, Educational and Industrial Testing Service, 1971.

29. Petty F, Noyes R: Depression secondary to cancer. Biol Psychiatry 16:1203-1220, 1981.

30. Derogatis LR, Morrow GR, Fetting J, et al: The prevalence of psychiatric disorders among cancer patients. JAMA 249:751-757, 1983.

31. Massie MJ, Holland JC: Diagnosis and treatment of depression in the cancer patient. J Clin Psychiatry 45:25-29, 1984.

32. Plumb M, Holland JC: Comparative studies of psychological function in patients with advanced cancer. II. Interviewer-rated current and past psychological symptoms. Psychosom Med 43:243-254, 1981.

33. Andersen BL, Hacker NF: Psychosexual adjustment after vulvar surgery. Obstet Gynecol 62:457-462, 1983.

34. Goldberg RJ, Wool MS, Glicksman A, et al: Relationship of the social environment and patients' physical status to depression in lung cancer patients and their spouses. J Psychosoc Oncol 2:73-80, 1984.

35. Metzger LF, Rogers TF, Bauman LJ: Effects of age and marital status on the emotional distress after a mastectomy. J Psychosoc Oncol 1:17-33, 1983.

36. Robinson JK, Boshier ML, Dansak DA, et al: Depression and anxiety in cancer patients: Evidence for different causes. J Psychosom Res 29:133-138, 1985.

37. Bukberg J, Penman D, Holland JC: Depression in hospitalized cancer patients. Psychosom Med 46:199-212, 1984.

38. Spitzer RL: Diagnostic and Statistical Manual of Mental Disorders-Revised (DSM-III-R). Washington, DC, American Psychiatric Association, 1987.

39. Layne C, Heitkemper T, Roehrig RA, Speer TK: Motivational deficit in depressed cancer patients. J Clin Psychol 41:139-144, 1985.

40. Morris T, Greer S, White P: Psychological and social adjustment to mastectomy: A two-year follow-up study. Cancer 40:2381-2387, 1977.

41. Beck AT, Lester D, Trexler L, et al: The measurement of pessimism: The hopelessness scale. J Consult Clin Psychol 42:861-865, 1974.

42. Nowotny ML: Assessment of hope in patients with cancer: Development of an instrument. Oncol Nurs Forum 16:57-61, 1989.

43. Herth KA: The relationship between level of hope and level of coping response and other variables in patients with cancer. Oncol Nurs Forum 16:67-72, 1989.

44. Schmale AH, Iker HP: The affect of hopelessness and the development of cancer. Psychosom Med 28:714-721, 1966.

45. Hinds PS: Adolescent hopefulness in illness and health. Adv Nurs Sci 10:79-88, 1988.

46. Dufault KJ: Hope of elderly persons with cancer (doctoral dissertation, Case Western Reserve University). Diss Abstr Intl 42:1820B, 1981.

47. Zook DJ, Yasko JM: Psychologic factors: Their effect on nausea and vomiting experiences by clients receiving chemotherapy. Oncol Nurs Forum 10:76-81, 1983.

48. Greene SM, O'Mahoney PD, Rungasamy P: Levels of measured hopelessness in physically-ill patients. J Psychosom Res 26:591-593, 1982.

49. Raleigh ED: An investigation of hope as manifested in the physically ill adult (doctoral dissertation, Wayne State University). Diss Abstr Intl 41:1313B, 1980.

50. Brandt B: The relationship between hopelessness and selected variables in women receiving chemotherapy for breast cancer. Oncol Nurs Forum 14:35-39, 1987.

51. Stoner M: Hope and cancer patients (doctoral dissertation, University of Colorado Health Sciences Center). Diss Abstr Intl 44:115-B, 1982.

52. Stoner M, Keampfer S: Recalled life expectancy information, phase of illness, and hope in cancer patients. Res Nurs Health 8:269-274, 1985.

53. Cassileth BR, Zupkis RV, Sutton-Smith K, et al: Information and participation preferences among cancer patients. Ann Intern Med 92:832-836, 1980.

54. Kerber A: Locus of control, hope, and disease-free interval (unpublished master's thesis), Emory University, Atlanta, Ga, 1985.

55. Clark JC: Hope as a critical factor in the cancer experience, in Pritchard AP (ed): Cancer Nursing: A Revolution in Care, Proceeding of the Fifth International Conference on Cancer Nursing. London, Macmillan, 1989, pp 117-119.

56. Dufault K, Martocchio BC: Hope: Its spheres and dimensions. Nurs Clin North Am 20:379-391, 1985.

57. Derogatis LR: Psychological assessment of psychosexual function. Psychiatr Clin North Am 3:113-131, 1980.

58. Waterhouse J, Metcalfe MC: Development of the sexual adjustment questionnaire. Oncol Nurs Forum 13:53-59, 1986.

59. Abitbol MM, Davenport JH: Sexual dysfunction after therapy for cervical carcinoma. Am J Obstet Gynecol 119:181-189, 1974.

60. Jenkins B: Patients' reports of sexual changes after treatment for gynecological cancer. Oncol Nurs Forum 15:349-354, 1988.

61. Cain EN, Kohorn EI, Quinlan DM, et al: Psychosocial reactions to the diagnosis of gynecologic cancer. Obstet Gynecol 62:635-641, 1983.

62. Andersen BL, Hacker NF: Psychosexual adjustment after vulvar surgery. Obstet Gynecol 62:457-462, 1983.

63. Andreasson B, Moth I, Jensen SB, et al: Sexual function and somatopsychic reactions in vulvectomy-operated women and their partners. Acta Obstet Gynecol Scand 65:7-10, 1986.

64. Woods NF, Earp JA: Women with cured breast cancer. Nurs Res 27:279-285, 1978.

65. Jamison KR, Wellisch DK, Pasnau RO: Psychosocial aspects of mastectomy. I. The woman's perspective. Am J Psychiatry 135:432-436, 1978.

66. Taylor SE, Lichtman RR, Wood JV, et al: Illness-related and treatment-related factors in psychological adjustment to breast cancer. Cancer 55:2506-2513, 1985.

67. Blackmore C: The impact of orchidectomy upon the sexuality of the man with testicular cancer. Cancer Nurs 11:33-40, 1988.

68. Schover LR, Gonzales M, von Eschenbach AC: Sexual and marital relationships after radiotherapy for seminoma. Urology 27:117-123, 1986.

69. Heinrich-Rynning T: Prostatic cancer treatments and their effects on sexual functioning. Oncol Nurs Forum 14:37-41, 1987.

70. Banker FL: The preservation of potency after external beam

irradiation for prostate cancer. Int J Radiat Oncol Biol Phys 15:219-220, 1988.

71. Labenne WD, Greene BI: Educational Implications of the Self-Concept Theory. Goodyear Publishing Company, 1969, p 10.

72. Newman KA, Schnaper N, Reed WP, et al: Effect of Hickman catheters on the self-esteem of patients with leukemia. South Med J 77:682-685, 1984.

73. Crumbaugh JC: Cross validation of purpose-in-life test based on Frankl's concepts. J Individual Psychol 24:74-81, 1968.

74. Weddington WW, Segraves KB, Simon MA: Psychological outcome of extremity sarcoma survivors undergoing amputation or limb salvage. J Clin Oncol 3:1393-1399, 1985.

75. Baxley KO, Erdman LK, Henry EB, et al: Alopecia: Effect on cancer patients' body image. Cancer Nurs 7:499-503, 1984.

76. Jourard S, Secord PF: Body cathexis and personality. Br J Psychol 46:130-138, 1955.

77. Kemeny MM, Wellisch DK, Schain WS: Psychosocial outcome in a randomized surgical trial for treatment of primary breast cancer. Cancer 62:1231-1237, 1988.

78. Annon JS: The Behavioral Treatment of Sexual Problems (vol 1). Honolulu, Mercentile Printing, 1974.

79. Lamb MA, Woods NF: Sexuality and the cancer patient. Cancer Nurs 4:137-144, 1981.

80. Shipes E, Lehr S: Sexuality and the male cancer patient. Cancer Nurs 5:375-381, 1982.

81. Capone MA, Good RS, Westie KS, et al: Psychosocial rehabilitation of gynecologic oncology patients. Arch Phys Med Rehabil 61:128-132, 1980.

82. Cain EN, Kohorn EI, Quinlan DM, et al: Psychosocial reactions to the diagnosis of gynecologic cancer. Obstet Gynecol 62:635-641, 1983.

Chapter 18

Psychosocial Dimensions: The Family

Jane Clark, RN, MN, OCN

INTRODUCTION

The diagnosis of cancer, although assigned to the individual, can precipitate significant changes in the lives of the individual, members of the family unit, and community. Although responses experienced vary among family members, across developmental stages of the family, with different illness demands, and with respect to economic and psychosocial resources, anecdotal data and clinical observations have substantiated the theoretical assumption that a change in one element of the social system, in this case the patient diagnosed with cancer, will result in a ripple effect throughout the system.

Predictability with respect to family routines, relationships, and communication patterns is threatened. Family members are challenged to learn new roles, self-care skills, and ways of relating and communicating to each other, friends, and members of the health care team as they cope with the chronic nature of the cancer experience. Life for families facing cancer becomes more complex. Although the demands of family members may be increased, few empirical studies have been conducted to describe the psychosocial responses of the family unit or individual members of the family unit to the cancer experience.[1]

Selected clinical and research instruments for evaluating the family will be described in this chapter. In addition, representative studies describing the responses of family members to the cancer experience, factors that place the family unit at risk for extreme responses, and effectiveness of selected interventions to modify responses of family members will be examined.

INSTRUMENTS TO EVALUATE THE FAMILY

The Family APGAR[2] is a screening questionnaire designed to assess family Adaptability, Partnership, Growth, Affection, and Resolve from the perspective of the patient. The questionnaire consists of five questions to which the patient responds on a 3-point scale indicating the frequency of satisfaction on the dimensions measured (almost always = 2; some of the time = 1; or hardly ever = 0). Based on the definition of family as a "psychosocial group consisting of the patient and one or more persons, children or adults, in which there is a commitment for members to nurture each other" (p. 1232), the instrument does not assume the structural, institutional, or cultural boundaries of the traditional family. Reliability and validity data were not reported by the author.

The Family Functioning Index (FFI)[3] is a 15-item self-report instrument designed to assess the dynamics of family interaction. Questions assess areas of marital satisfaction, frequency of disagreement, communication, problem solving, and feelings of happiness and closeness.[4] Validity and reliability estimates for the instrument were determined by comparing scores on the FFI with clinical ratings by caseworkers and by resulting high positive correlations of husband and wife scores. Five-year test-retest reliability was reported as $r = .83$, $p < .001$.[4]

RESPONSES OF THE FAMILY TO PHASES OF THE CANCER EXPERIENCE

In the previous chapter, the individual responses of anxiety, depression, hopelessness, and altered sexual health were discussed with respect to the diagnosis of cancer. Surprisingly, the responses of family members have been shown to be similar to those of patients with cancer.

Responses of Family Members in General

Self-reported responses of family members to hospitalization of patients with cancer were described by Lovejoy.[5] Data were obtained from 105 subjects using a semistructured interview schedule. Content analyses of the interviews revealed five common responses to the hospitalization experience: shock, uncertainty, accommodation, immersion, and awareness. The responses were not unlike patient responses described by other researchers.

A comparison of psychological responses of patients with cancer and their next-of-kin ($N = 210$) was reported by Cassileth et al.[6] Patient and next-of-kin scores on three outcome measures—State-Trait Anxiety Inventory, Profile of Mood States, and Mental Health Index—were correlated significantly. Scores for both patients and next-of-kin indicated a decrease in psychological status related to the phase of the cancer experience; that is, the psychological status was better for patients and next-of-kin during follow-up care versus active treatment versus palliative care.

Responses of Spouses

Findings of Casselith et al[6] were supported by Oberst and James[7] in a study to determine the magnitude and pattern of crisis development among spouses of cancer patients ($N = 40$), to describe the effectiveness of crisis counseling, and to identify factors that predict crisis development (p. 48). Findings indicated that spouses experienced increased anxiety before the patient was discharged from the hospital, which was replaced by depression and anger at patients for egocentricity in the home care period. Depression and anger were succeeded eventually by guilt. Moreover, spouses reported distress, anger, and frustration about the lack of support from professionals and all sources (p. 56). Spouses also had a higher incidence of emotional problems than did the patients at 10, 30, 60, 90, and 180 days after discharge. In addition to the psychological responses to the demands of

TABLE 18-1 Perceived Spousal Caregiving Demands

Management of physical care

Management of household finances

Standing by

Alterations in caregiver's well-being and pattern of living

Unmet expectations from the health care system

Constant vigilance

Cancer

Anticipation of the future

Alterations in relationship with ill spouse

Source: Stetz KM: Caregiving demands during advanced cancer: The spouse's needs. Cancer Nurs 10(5):260-268, 1987.

TABLE 18-2 Psychosocial Problems Experienced by Family Members

Impaired relationships with the family or significant others

Impaired relationships with health care providers

Somatic side effects of disease and treatment

Difficulties in compliance with treatment

Mood disturbances

Difficulties in family roles

Difficulties in self-management

Financial difficulties

Transportation difficulties

Equipment difficulties

Significant concerns about body image

Denial

Cognitive impairment

Source: Wellisch DK, Fawzy FI, Landsverk J, et al: Evaluation of psychosocial problems of the home-bound cancer patient: The relationship of disease and the sociodemographic variables of patients to family problems. J Psychosoc Oncol 1:4-5, 1983.

the cancer experience, spouses reported disruption in many areas of lifestyle, including employment, home management, child care, social activities, and travel to and from hospital. Thus, the acute hospitalization period precipitates significant psychological responses among spouses of patients with cancer that continue through the postdischarge home care period and even into the terminal phase of illness.

The findings of Oberst and James[7] were extended to the terminal phase of illness in a study by Stetz[8] of 65 spouses of terminally ill adult cancer patients. Content analyses of semistructured interviews conducted in the home revealed nine categories of spouse caregiving demands (Table 18-1).[8] Gender differences were identified. Female caregivers had more difficulty with observing the physical deterioration of the spouse while male caregivers had more difficulty with home management.

The responses of spouses to home care demands were described by Wellisch et al.[9] Records of 447 homebound, married cancer patients were reviewed to determine the types of psychosocial problems experienced by family members (p. 1). A standardized instrument to abstract the frequencies of psychosocial problem areas (Table 18-2)[9] was used for review. Findings indicated that families of male patients were more likely to feel overwhelmed by the demands of home care ($p = .0003$) and were more likely to experience a severe mood disturbance ($p = .0001$) than were families of female patients.

Age had a significant impact on the family variables studied. Families of patients 70 years or older were more likely to be overwhelmed by home care demands ($p = .0311$). Role disturbances were more likely to occur in families of patients age 50 years or younger ($p = .04$), while mood disturbances were more likely to occur in families of patients 50 years or older ($p = .02$).

The findings of the study indicated that the type of cancer diagnosed, that is, lung, breast, or cervical cancer, had a specific impact on family outcome variables. The

families of patients with lung cancer were more likely to exhibit significant mood disturbances ($p = .001$) and to be overwhelmed by the demands of home care ($p = .003$). In contrast, families of patients with cervical cancer were more likely to experience disturbances in family relationships ($p = .01$).

The findings of Goldberg et al[10] support the high incidence of depression among spouses (N = 18) of patients with lung cancer. Scores on the Profile of Mood States-Depression were measured within 6 weeks of diagnosis and at 2-month intervals for a total of 6 months. Spouses had elevated mean scores at diagnosis (Time 1 = 14.7), and the mean scores remained elevated throughout the data-collection period (Time 2 = 11.3, Time 3 = 10.6). In addition, scores of spouses on the Psychosocial Adjustment to Illness Scale (social environment subscale) were related significantly to the depression scores rather than to the physical status scores of the patient at all three time intervals.

Other psychosocial responses of spouses of patients with lung cancer were described by Cooper.[11] Fifteen patients with lung cancer and their spouses were interviewed to determine the effects of the diagnosis on the family. In content analyses of the interviews, the following effects were identified. Spouses experienced shock, fear, and depression at diagnosis. Spouses also reported more symptoms of stress (nervousness, sleeplessness, loss of appetite, inability to concentrate, and irritability) than did patients. Moreover, spouses reported feelings of aloneness and helplessness in response to the cancer experience.

Communication patterns between the patient-spouse dyads changed in that the spouses became protective of the patient with respect to discussing distressful information and reported not sharing their feelings with patients. Despite changed communication patterns, the majority of subjects reported increased closeness in patient-spouse and parent-child relationships.

Northouse and Northouse[12] reviewed 200 clinical papers and research studies printed over two decades to identify issues of communication among patients, health care professionals, and family members. The authors argue that although the number of articles on communication issues among family members of persons with cancer is limited, the potential impact of communication issues on the care of the patient and the well-being of family members is far-reaching.

Communication becomes a primary issue among family members as caregiving demands increase. Data indicate that although the responsibilities of care are being shifted to the family, family members express concern over the difficulty in obtaining necessary information.[13-15] Second, as the demands of care increase, mood disturbances among family members, particularly anxiety and depression,[7,16,17] become more prominent. However, professional concern for care of family members has been limited, and family members have not communicated their concerns and responses to health care professionals.

Responses of Adult and Adolescent Children

Just as data indicate that communication patterns can become strained between the patient and spouse facing cancer, indications are that communication patterns change between the parents and children within the family. Lichtman et al[18] interviewed 78 patients with a diagnosis of breast cancer to describe changes in the relationships between patients and their children and to examine the factors that influence these changes. In addition to structured interviews, the subjects completed the Profile of Mood States, Self-Esteem Scale,[19] Index of Well-Being,[20] and Marital Adjustment Scale.[21] Patients were also asked to provide the name of a significant other to be interviewed ($N = 63$).

Findings indicated 54% of patients ($N = 37$) reported changes in the relationships with children. The changes were characterized as improved (73%) and permanent (76%). Nineteen problem relationships were identified. Patients attributed the problems to changes in how the children were responding to the patient (28%) and how the patients were responding to the children (10%), changes in both response patterns (52%), and changes due to other reasons (10%). These findings were confirmed by interviews with identified significant others.

Deteriorated relationships were correlated significantly with a poor prognosis for the patient ($r = .32$, $p<.02$) as well as the severity of surgery ($r = .43$, $p<.001$). In addition, patient adjustment scores were predictive of perceived changes in relationships with children ($r = .20$, $p<.05$) in that patients with poor adjustment scores reported more changes and negative changes in relationships with children.

Changes in relationships with children differed significantly with respect to the gender of the child ($x^2(1) = 3.92$, $p<.05$). Although patients reported similar problems with fears related to prognosis, rejection, and refusal to discuss cancer in both mother-son and mother-daughter relationships, the frequency and magnitude of the problems were greater in the mother-daughter relationships.

The relationships with adult children can become more complex when the adult child is a health care professional. In a cross-sectional study by Baird[22] of 27 nurse/daughters, the subjects were interviewed and asked to compare their perceptions of family relationships before and after the diagnosis of cancer. Nurse/daughter perceptions of roles changed with the diagnosis of cancer in the following ways: roles expanded from that of information source to decision maker, intermediary, and caregiver. Even though the role changes were perceived as positive, nurse/daughters described role conflicts between daughter/nurse, sibling/nurse, and family member/nurse. However, positive changes in communication patterns were identified by 59% of the sample. Parents and family members were perceived to be more open, closer, and dependent after the diagnosis of cancer.

Loss of a parent during adolescence has been documented as a critical event in the life of a child. Berman et al[23] interviewed 10 adolescents and the surviving parent within 6 months to 2 years following the death of a parent of cancer to describe responses experienced. The adolescents described open information sharing among the family unit during the illness; however, after the death, communication patterns changed. The adolescent reportedly assumed the protector role in shielding the remaining parent from discussing distressful feelings. The adolescents, as did the spouses in the previous studies, indicated that the protector role was extremely stressful and that they lacked sufficient support during this period.

Discrepancies were reported between parents and adolescents in the changes in activities of daily living as well as in the sources of support for the adolescents. Adolescents perceived an increase in household responsibilities as well as more support from family and peers versus health care professionals and clergy.

EFFECT OF FAMILY RESPONSES ON PATTERNS AND OUTCOMES OF CARE

Whereas the majority of studies in the area of family responses to a diagnosis of cancer have been to describe the responses experienced in families of selected patient groups (site-specific or age-specific), limited data exist to quantify the impact of those responses on either outcomes or patterns of care. Hays[24] conducted a retrospective chart review of visits to 100 patients with cancer during the last 10 days of their lives to determine if the incidence of symptoms, family coping, and resources used were predictive of home and inpatient hospice use. The random sample of home care patients (group I, home care only; group II, home care/inpatient) were evaluated on physical symptoms of pain, nausea, vomiting, respiratory deficit, elimination, nutrition, and mental status; family coping patterns of anxiety and fatigue; and patterns of care including length and frequency of home visits, disciplines visited, telephone contacts, home care episodes, and place of death.

Patients who experienced more physical symptoms and more symptoms that were uncontrolled were more likely to require inpatient hospice services. Uncontrolled symptoms associated with increased anxiety and fatigue experienced by family members and demand for homecare services also increased the use of inpatient hospice services.

The relationships of family cohesion and adaptability (FACES II),[25] marital adjustment (Snyder Marital Disharmony and Disaffection Scales),[26] and psychosocial adjustment to illness (Psychosocial Adjustment to Illness Scale)[27] among 57 white women with breast cancer were explored by Friedman et al.[28] Based on the theoretical framework proposed by Olson et al,[29] the researchers examined if women who perceived that their families were balanced rather than extreme with respect to emotional connectedness and flexibility to change reported more positive levels of adjustment.

Findings supported the notion that family cohesion is a desirable quality among women faced with a diagnosis of breast cancer. In fact, 34% of the respondents expressed a desire for more cohesiveness within the family, while no respondent indicated that she desired less cohesiveness. Data analyses revealed that women who reported the highest levels of family cohesion also reported more positive adjustment to breast cancer. No significant relationship was found between reported family adaptability and adjustment to breast cancer. Although the findings are not consistent with the propositions of the model offered by Olsen et al,[29] the authors question if gender differences with respect to value of affection versus task orientation could have contributed to the differences seen in the study sample.

ASSESSMENT CRITERIA

The family is identified as a portion of four nursing diagnoses identified by the North American Nursing Diagnosis Association (NANDA): (1) Alteration in family processes, (2) Ineffective family coping: compromised, (3) Ineffective family coping: disabling, and (4) Family coping: potential for growth.[30] A comparison of each diagnosis is presented in Table 18-3.

The complexities of assessment measures of the family are detailed by Lewis.[1] Yet, the complexities of measures only reflect the complexities of the phenomena of study, in this case the family coping with the cancer experience. Thus the ideal assessment of families using multiple measures from multiple sources described by Lewis[1] offer the potential for collecting the most comprehensive and reliable data base on which to base family-level services.

However, the personnel and time demanded by such an extensive assessment precludes application to all families in the clinical setting. Yet, screening instruments described previously may serve to identify those families at high risk for dysfunctional responses to the cancer experience and to target families in need of a more comprehensive assessment.

FAMILY-LEVEL NURSING INTERVENTIONS

Selection of nursing interventions for families facing cancer is based on the needs of the individual family members as well as the needs expressed by the family unit. Family-level teaching with respect to the disease, treatment, rehabilitation, or prognosis; anticipatory guidance of family members throughout the cancer experience; single and multiple family group counseling; mobilization of health care or community resources; and referrals for intensive family therapy have been identified in the literature as strategies for family care.[31-35]

Although nursing interventions may be directed toward the individual members or the family unit, the majority of studies among families facing cancer have focused on the individual family members. Few empirical studies have been conducted to determine the effects of family-unit services. The effects of selected interventions on family outcomes will be discussed in the following section.

Spousal Support Groups

Sabo et al[36] studied the responses of husbands of 24 patients who had undergone a mastectomy ($N = 24$) and the effects of a 10-week support group intervention ($N = 6$) in modifying those responses. All subjects were interviewed and completed a 37-item self-report instrument to evaluate gender expectations, self-esteem, depression, sexual compatibility, frequency of verbal communication about the mastectomy, and supportive attitude toward the wife before the intervention. Six husbands elected to attend the support group.

Interview findings indicated that the husbands had strong reactions of disbelief, alarm, isolation, and anxiety related to the role of support-giver for the wife. After the surgery, the husbands described assuming the role of protector to shield the wife from both his and her emotional reactions to the cancer experience, which resulted in strained communication patterns, distrust, and resentment. Comparison of pre and post scores on the instrument revealed that husbands who had attended the support group communicated significantly more with their wives about mastectomy issues than did husbands who had not attended the group sessions.

TABLE 18-3 Comparison of Family-Related Nursing Diagnoses

Nursing Diagnosis	Definition	Defining Characteristics
Alteration in Family Processes	Inability of family system (household members) to meet needs of members, carry out family functions, or maintain communications for mutual growth and maturation	Inability of family members to relate to each other for mutual growth and maturation, failure to send and receive clear messages, poorly communicated family rules, rituals, symbols, unexplained myths, unhealthy family decision-making processes, inability of family members to express and accept wide range of feelings, inability to accept and receive help, does not demonstrate respect for individuality and autonomy of members, rigidity in functions and roles, fails to accomplish current or past family developmental tasks, inappropriate boundary maintenance, inability to adapt to change, inability to deal with traumatic or crisis experience constructively, parents do not demonstrate respect for each other's views on child-rearing practices, inappropriate level and direction of energy, inability to meet needs of members, family uninvolved in community activities
Ineffective Family Coping: Compromised	Usually supportive primary person providing insufficient, ineffective, or compromised support, comfort, assistance, or encouragement that may be needed by patient to manage or master adaptive tasks related to health challenge	Patient expresses concern or complaint about significant other's response to health problem, significant persons described preoccupation with personal reactions to patient's illness, disability, or other situational or developmental crisis, significant person describes or confirms inadequate understanding of knowledge base which interferes with effective assistive or supportive behaviors, significant person attempts assistive or supportive behaviors with less than satisfactory results, significant person withdraws or enters into a limited or temporary personal communication with client at time of need, significant person displays protective behavior disproportionate to patient's abilities or need for autonomy
Ineffective Family Coping: Disabled	Behavior of significant person disables own capabilities and patient's capacities to address effectively tasks essential to either person's adaptation to the health challenge	Neglectful care of patient in regard to basic human needs and/or illness treatment, distortion of reality regarding patient's health problem including extreme denial, intolerance, rejection, abandonment, desertion, carrying on usual routines disregarding patient needs, psychosomaticism, taking on illness signs of the patient, decisions or actions by family which are detrimental to economic or social well-being, agitation, depression, aggression, hostility, impaired restructuring of a meaningful life for self, impaired individuation, prolonged overconcern for patient, neglectful relationships with other family members, patient's development of helpless, inactive dependence
Family Coping: Potential for Growth	Family member has managed adaptive tasks involved with patient's health challenge effectively and is exhibiting desire and readiness for enhanced health and growth in regard to self and in relation to the patient	Family member attempts to describe growth impact of crisis on his/her own values, priorities, goals, or relationships, is moving in direction of health-promoting and enriching lifestyle which supports and monitors maturational processes, audits and negotiated treatment program and generally chooses experiences which optimize wellness, expresses interest in making contact on a one-to-one basis or on a mutual-aid group basis with another person who has experienced a similar situation

Source: Gordon M: Manual of Nursing Diagnosis 1986-1987. New York, McGraw-Hill, 1987.

Risk Counseling Interventions

To address the need of family members for information about the cancer of the patient as well as personal risks for cancer, Kelly[37] described a program of risk counseling designed specifically for relatives of persons with cancer. Based on the expressed concerns of the relative, elements of the program may include biologic and medical information about cancer risks or a review of individual personality, life-style, and environmental risks. In addition, relatives may be counseled on how to deal with tensions in the family, how to express concern for the family member with cancer, and how to deal with personal physical and psychosocial responses to the cancer experience. Data related to the outcomes of the program were not reported by the author.

FUTURE DIRECTIONS FOR NURSING RESEARCH

The issues of family responses to a diagnosis of cancer go far beyond those discussed in the previous chapter. Even though selected psychosocial responses have been identified for spouses, patient–significant other dyads, and children of adults with cancer, the effects of the interaction of those individual responses within the context of the family unit have not been studied systematically. The lack of data becomes even more critical when one considers the responses of nontraditional family units, multigenerational families, and culturally diverse families.

Obviously, family-level services are not needed nor available for every family faced with cancer. However, screening instruments with established reliability and validity among families facing cancer and delineation of critical defining characteristics that predispose the family to dysfunctional responses are areas requiring additional study.

Finally, given the identification of high-risk or dysfunctional families, individual and family-level services to address expressed dysfunctional responses among cancer families are minimal. Multiple services and programs designed to meet a spectrum of family needs are needed. In addition, the effectiveness of such services and programs in modifying the occurrence or resolution of dysfunctional responses in the family must be evaluated.

REFERENCES

1. Lewis FM: Family level services for the cancer patient: Critical distinctions, fallacies, and assessment. Cancer Nurs 6:193-200, 1983.
2. Smilkstein G: The family APGAR: A proposal for a family function test and its use by physicians. J Family Pract 6:1231-1239, 1978.
3. Pless IB, Satterwhite BB: A measure of family functioning and its application. Soc Sci Med 7:613-620, 1973.
4. Satterwhite BB, Zweig SR, Iker HP, et al: The family functioning index—five-year test-retest reliability and implications for use. J Comp Family Studies 7:111-116, 1976.
5. Lovejoy NC: Family responses to cancer hospitalization. Oncol Nurs Forum 13:33-37, 1986.
6. Cassileth BR, Lusk EJ, Strouse TB, et al: A psychological analysis of cancer patients and their next-of-kin. Cancer 55:72-76, 1985.
7. Oberst MT, James RH: Going home: Patient and spouse adjustment following cancer surgery. Topics Clin Nurs 7:46-57, 1985.
8. Stetz KM: Caregiving demands during advanced cancer: The spouse's needs. Cancer Nurs 10:260-268, 1987.
9. Wellisch DK, Fawzy FI, Landsverk J, et al: Evaluation of psychosocial problems of the home-bound cancer patient: The relationship of disease and the sociodemographic variables of patients to family problems. J Psychosoc Oncol 1:1-15, 1983.
10. Goldberg RJ, Wool MS, Glicksman A, et al: Relationship of the social environment and patients' physical status to depression in lung cancer patients and their spouses. J Psychosoc Oncol 2:73-80, 1984.
11. Cooper ET: A pilot study on the effects of the diagnosis of lung cancer on family relationships. Cancer Nurs 7:301-308, 1984.
12. Northouse PG, Northouse LL: Communication and cancer: Issues confronting patients, health professionals, and family members. J Psychosoc Oncol 5:17-46, 1987.
13. Krant MJ, Johnston L: Family members' perceptions of communication in late stage cancer. Int J Psychiatry Med 8:203-216, 1977-1978.
14. Morrow GR, Hoagland AC, Morse IP: Sources of support perceived by parents of children with cancer: Implications for counseling. Patient Counsel Health Ed 4:36-40, 1982.
15. Wright K, Dyck S: Expressed concerns of adult cancer patients' family members. Cancer Nurs 7:371-374, 1984.
16. Baider L, Kaplan De-Nour A, Atara K: Couples' reactions and adjustment to mastectomy: A preliminary report. Int J Psychiatry Med 14:265-276, 1984.
17. Northouse LL: The impact of cancer on the family: An overview. Int J Psychiatry Med 14:215-242, 1984.
18. Lichtman RR, Taylor SE, Wood JV, et al: Relations with children after breast cancer: The mother-daughter relationship at risk. J Psychosoc Oncol 2:1-19, 1984.
19. Rosenberg M: Society and the Adolescent Self-Image. Princeton, NJ, Princeton University Press, 1965.
20. Campbell A, Converse PE, Rodgers WL: The Quality of American Life: Perceptions, Evaluations, and Satisfactions. New York, Russell Sage Foundation, 1976.
21. Locke HF, Wallace KM: Short marital adjustment and prediction tests: Their reliability and validity. Marriage Family Living 21:251-255, 1959.
22. Baird SB: The effect of cancer in a parent on role relationships with the nurse/daughter. Cancer Nurs 11:9-17, 1988.
23. Berman H, Cragg CE, Kuenzig L: Having a parent die of cancer: Adolescents' reactions. Oncol Nurs Forum 15:159-162, 1988.
24. Hays JC: Patient symptoms and family coping: Predictors of hospice utilization patterns. Cancer Nurs 9:317-325, 1986.
25. Olson DH, Portner J, Bell R: Family Adaptability and Cohesion Evaluation Scales (FACES II). St. Paul, University of Minnesota, Family Social Science, 1982.
26. Snyder DK, Regts JM: Factor scales for assessing marital disharmony and disaffection. J Consult Clin Psychol 50:736-743, 1982.
27. Derogatis LR, Lopez MC: The Psychosocial Adjustment to Illness Scale (PAIS & PAIS-SR): Administration, Scoring, and

Procedures Manual-I. Baltimore, Md, Johns Hopkins University School of Medicine, 1983.

28. Friedman LC, Baer PE, Nelson DV, et al: Women with breast cancer: Perception of family functioning and adjustment to illness. Psychosom Med 50:529-540, 1988.

29. Olson DH, Sprenkle DH, Russell CS: Circumplex model of marital and family systems. I. Cohesion and adaptability dimensions, family types and clinical applications. Family Process 18:3-28, 1979.

30. Gordon M: Manual of Nursing Diagnosis 1986-1987. New York, McGraw-Hill, 1987.

31. Whitman HH, Gustafson JP: Group therapy for families facing a cancer crisis. Oncol Nurs Forum 16:539-543, 1989.

32. Giacquinta B: Helping families face the crisis of cancer. Am J Nurs 77:1585-1588, 1977.

33. Wellisch DK, Mosher MB, Van Scoy C: Management of family emotion stress: Family group therapy in a private oncology practice. Int J Group Psychother 28:225-231, 1978.

34. Edstrom S, Woehning Miller MW: Preparing the family to care for the cancer patient at home: A home care course. Cancer Nurs 4:49-52, 1981.

35. Heinricks RL, Coscarelli Schag C: Stress and activity management: Group treatment for cancer patients and spouses. J Consult Clin Psychol 53:439-446, 1985.

36. Sabo D, Brown J, Smith C: The male role and mastectomy: Support groups and men's adjustment. J Psychosoc Oncol 4:19-31, 1986.

37. Kelly PT: Risk counseling for relatives of cancer patients: New information, new approaches. J Psychosoc Oncol 5:65-79, 1987.

Chapter 19

Psychosocial Dimensions: Issues in Survivorship

Deborah Welch-McCaffrey, RN, MSN, OCN

Susan Leigh, RN, BSN

Lois J. Loescher, RN, MS

Barbara Hoffman, JD

INTRODUCTION

Early detection and effective multimodal therapies have increased significantly the numbers of cancer survivors to the extent that cancer is now considered a chronic, life-threatening illness rather than a terminal disease.[1] In 1989, over 5 million Americans had a history of cancer, with 3 million surviving 5 years or more.[2] Cancers with a high and continually increasing 5-year relative survival rate include testicular cancer (86%), endometrial cancer (85%), cutaneous melanoma (80%), breast cancer (74%), bladder cancer (73%), Hodgkin's disease (73%), prostate cancer (70%), and cervical cancer (67%).[2,3]

The health care community traditionally has been more concerned with the aggressive medical treatment of patients having cancers with a high survival rate than with the psychosocial aspects of long-term survivorship.[4] The burgeoning population of survivors, however, makes evident the need to address quality of survival and the psychosocial consequences of cancer and its therapies. Long-term survivors may experience problems ranging from minor short-term difficulties to major psychosocial crises.[5-7] Determining which individuals are at greatest risk for psychosocial morbidity is critical for clinicians.

DEFINITIONS OF SURVIVORSHIP

Survivorship as defined by *Webster's Ninth New Collegiate Dictionary* is summarized as the state of remaining alive or in existence (living on) and continuing to function or prosper despite life occurrences.[8] Medical definitions of long-term cancer survivorship are more limited in scope and are not yet fully agreed on by the health care community. Historically, cancer survivors have been defined as individuals "cured" of their disease, with the "cured" state commencing 5 years after diagnosis.[2] The term *cure* traditionally describes those individuals who have no evidence of disease with a minimal or nonexistent chance for recurrence.[9]

Controversial aspects of associating survivorship with cancer "cure" could be eliminated by basing the definition on the concept of control rather than "cure." Cancer itself constitutes many different diseases, each having distinct stages and behaviors and treated with a wide range of modalities. Some cancers, such as melanoma or early stages of breast cancer, are often "cured" once the cancer is physically removed. Other cancers, including stage I and stage II Hodgkin's disease, acute lymphocytic leukemias, and osteogenic sarcoma, may be considered cured following several courses of intensive multimodal therapy.[10] Individuals with these types of cancers may be, by definition, "cured" before the fifth year following diagnosis, but they are still not medically considered cured and, thus, a long-term survivor until the 5-year mark. Still other cancers such as multiple myeloma or chronic leukemia may not be "curable" but, with continued treatment, can be controlled, enabling patients to live for several years. Although these individuals are not "cured" in the medical sense, they are indeed survivors of a chronic disease. Finally, other cancers are initially labelled "incurable" or advanced at diagnosis, with expectations of inevitable death.[11] Exceptional patients who survive these cancers may be defined further as "miracle cures."

Vought et al[12] described a survival paradigm that allows health care providers to rank the importance of the issues a survivor might identify.[13] The six components of the paradigm are listed in descending order of importance but not in order of occurrence: (1) basic survival (food, shelter, medical care); (2) physiologic self-concept (attractiveness, fitness, physical function); (3) psychologic self-concept (self-respect, integrity, autonomy); (4) proximal affiliation (intimate relationships); (5) distal affiliation (social relationships); and (6) avocational component (recreation and play). Cancer-related barriers to the survival paradigm are listed in Table 19-1. Although physical self-concept has a higher importance rating, psychosocial components comprise the bulk of the model, indicating the overall importance of psychosocial issues.

SURVIVORSHIP AS A CONTINUUM

Using the control definition enables cancer survivorship to be viewed as a continual, ongoing process rather than as an explicit event occurring at a predetermined time period. Mullan[14] first proposed a continuum of survival stages or "seasons" in lieu of the word "cure." Seasons of survival apply to everyone diagnosed with cancer and consist of an acute, extended, and permanent survival stage. The acute survival stage begins at diagnosis, when patients must deal with immediate effects of therapy in addition to their mortality. Life modifications that will become part of their immediate and long-term future are begun. Social support of the patient is critical in this stage. Extended survival begins when the patient's disease has gone into remission or the patient has finished the primary treatment course and starts consolidation or adjuvant therapies. In this stage, patients begin to deal with issues such as altered body image or vocational changes. Psychosocial treatment is often lacking in the extended survival stage. Finally, Mullan[14] described the permanent survival stage that is most frequently associated with "cure" and evolves from the time when cancer activity or the chance of its return decreases and the disease can be arrested permanently. Economic problems often surface in this stage, along with concern for long-term and late effects of cancer treatment. This chapter will concentrate on psychosocial issues prevalent in the extended and permanent survival stages.

Agreement on a definition of survivorship will enable the adaptation or development of other survivorship models. Viewing cancer survivorship as an evolving process allows recognition of the fact that psychosocial issues of

TABLE 19-1 Components of a Cancer Survival Paradigm

Focus	Critical Elements	Cancer-Related Barrier
Basic survival	Concern about resources for food, shelter, medical care	Limited finances, loss of job benefits, lack of adequate follow-up medical care
Physical self-concept	Physical attractiveness, fitness, maintenance of body function	Any body image alteration, energy reserve impairment, residual physical disability
Psychological self-concept	Self-respect, integrity, autonomy	Use of self-blame, dependency, self-doubt, change in pre-cancer life-style
Proximal affiliation	Relationships with family, lovers, and close friends	Fears about hereditary transmission, family stress related to illness, alterations in customary social support, sexual dysfunction, concern about disclosure
Distal affiliation	Relationships to coworkers and acquaintances	Shunning and isolationism, discriminatory practices, concern about disclosure
Avocational	Recreation, play, escape	Physical compromise, financial constraints, fear of distancing self from health care team

Source: Reprinted by permission of the publisher from Vought CA, Dintruff DL, Fotopoulos SS: Adaptations to the constraints of cancer: Motivational issues, in Ahmed P(ed): Living and Dying with Cancer. New York, Elsevier, 1981, pp 205-219. Copyright 1981 by Elsevier Science Publishing Co, Inc.

long-term survivorship can arise in any stage or phase of the survival continuum. Thus, in anticipation of long-term survivorship, psychosocial interventions should begin at diagnosis, rather than when the patient is considered medically "cured."

PSYCHOSOCIAL THEMES

Survivorship encompasses many aspects of psychobiologic functioning. Studies confirm, however, a relative lack of psychopathology in long-term survivors of cancer.[5,15-20] The major psychosocial themes that can be anticipated in significant cohorts of adults surviving cancer are (1) interrelationships between physiologic long-term effects and psychosocial outcomes, (2) fears of relapse and death, (3) dependence on health care providers, (4) survivor guilt, (5) uncertain sense of longevity, (6) social adaptation dilemmas, and (7) contagion effect—the family as survivor.

Interrelationships Between Physiologic Long-Term Effects and Psychosocial Outcomes

An individual's ability to cope within the trajectory of extended or permanent survival can be strongly influenced by physiologic compromise.[14,21] In a study of 49 women 4 years after mastectomy, Woods and Earp[22] noted that subjects with more symptom distress associated with their surgery had greater degrees of depressive symptoms. Rieker

et al[23] studied 74 men 2 to 10 years after treatment for testicular cancer and found that those with resultant sexual impairment (ie, infertility, ejaculatory dysfunction) reported more psychologic symptomatology and strained intimate relationships than men without long-term sexual impairment. Fobair et al[6] noted the relationship of persistent energy loss and depression in 403 Hodgkin's disease survivors evaluated approximately 9 years after completion of therapy. Additional research that integrates the physical and psychosocial sequelae of surviving cancer will help identify those factors that enhance and detract from quality survival.

Fears of Relapse and Death

Probably the most common concern for all cancer survivors is the fear of cancer recurrence.[1,19,24-26] Not knowing when and if cancer will reappear often negatively affects the survivor's sense of control over his or her life.[27,28] Commonly referred to as the "Damocles syndrome," death anxiety often fluctuates in intensity as intermittent suspicious symptomatology is dealt with.[20] Fear of relapse may present in a variety of forms, ranging from general uneasiness about the etiology of mild to moderate somatic complaints to pronounced anxiety or panic attacks that interfere with daily life. Exaggerated worry over somatic distress is usually most intense within 2 years after completion of therapy.[4,24] As time passes, anxiety may lessen concerning relapse and recurrence. However, a heightened sense of vulnerability to illness is frequently a hallmark of the cancer survivor's long-term experience.[29]

Dependence on Health Care Providers

Both the survivor's need to determine the nature of suspicious symptomatology and the physician's need to evaluate the patient closely following cessation of therapy mandates an ongoing relationship between the patient and health care team. This reality often causes the patient to experience divergent reactions.

For many patients nearing the end of treatment, a significant ambivalence evolves. They are elated over the prospect of discontinuing therapy yet fear distancing themselves from the health care team who has helped them to get to this extended survival stage.[26,30] Mullan[25] also noted that the fear of recurrence along with the fear of the physician's finding disease can lead to behaviors such as hypochondriasis or avoidance of physicians. Routine checkups and yearly comprehensive examinations may engender pronounced anxiety.

Survivor Guilt

Waiting room scenarios may also poignantly depict the negative outcomes from cancer, closely followed by the introspection, "Will I end up that way, too?" The infrequently discussed phenomenon of survivor guilt may appear at this time as well.[31] As comparisons are made among patients, one may ponder, "Why am I doing well and they aren't?" Similar to questions arising around the time of initial diagnosis, attempts to justify "Why me?" or "Why not me?" may resurface. Hence, the survivor's ongoing involvement with follow-up care is characterized by mixed emotional reactions and multiple concerns.

Uncertain Sense of Longevity

Because of the prevailing perception that cancer results in a painful, lingering death, most patients' immediate reaction to the diagnosis is the expectation of a shortened lifespan. Once successful completion of therapy is achieved, hope for continued survival often supercedes thoughts of death. Many survivors, however, change their life-style as a reaction to the possibility of dying younger than expected.

A critical evaluation of life's meaning and priorities seems to take utmost importance. Survivors report greater appreciation of life and become more satisfied with life as a whole.[31] A significant value reassessment leads to heightened awareness of things taken for granted and lessened concern for the trivial. Mullan[14] characterized this phenomenon as "life re-kindled." This enhanced global acceptance of greater appreciation of life and improved quality of life for the present represent important secondary benefits of having survived cancer.

Social Adaptation Dilemmas

Attempts to minimize memories of the treatment experience and to "get on with life" are not often easy tasks for the survivor. The transition from a sick role to a healthy role can be compromised by persistent physical debility (despite cessation of therapy), negative expectations from within one's social support realm, personal concerns about one's ability to readjust, and social stigma. Shunning, a highly subjective phenomenon, may be a pervasive barrier to successful reorientation.[25]

Similar to the patient's ambivalent relationship with the health care team, confusing reactions to available social support may deter social adaptation. On the one hand, the survivor may not want to be treated like a patient, yet the survivor may also react negatively to withdrawal of the intense social support mobilized during the initial diagnosis phase.[26] Repeated explanations about one's health status to family, friends, acquaintances, employers, and insurors may drain the survivor's emotional responses. Constant scrutiny from these individuals can also be stressful. Dealing with relationships outside the immediate family unit becomes more difficult if internal family needs are not met successfully.

Contagion Effect—The Family as Survivor

A plethora of information exists about the plight of the family coping with the active phases of cancer. However, there is a paucity of information about families coping with extended or permanent survival.[32] Premorbid family style is an important assessment variable in determining postillness coping.[20] Even the most supportive family member is not immune to long-term psychologic stress throughout the extensive cancer continuum. The family's anxiety about the patient, that is, worry over potential relapse and unfavorable social situations, may be exhibited by overprotectiveness and pervasive anxiety. Marital discord and changes in sexual relationships can occur. Family members may not want to listen to or hear the survivor's concerns over potential relapse, since these can trigger their own sense of insecurity about continued long-term survival. Woods and Earp[22] identified the presence of "conversational isolationism" in families hesitant to discuss mutual concerns about the recurrence of cancer. As health care professionals acknowledge cancer as a family disease, they must be sensitive to the ramifications of survival for all members of the family unit.

EMPLOYMENT AND INSURANCE DISCRIMINATION

Many cancer survivors encounter ongoing socioeconomic impediments to full recovery. Concerns include regaining financial and work-related stability and maintaining medical insurance coverage. Access to insurance is usually through employment, but the issues of job discrimination and insurance-related problems are separate and complicated and therefore will be addressed individually.

Employment Discrimination

Survivors' employment problems can be attributed to three predominant myths about cancer: (1) cancer is a death sentence, (2) cancer is contagious, and (3) cancer survivors are an unproductive drain on the economy.[2,33-35] Meanwhile, current statistics indicate that more than half of all Americans diagnosed with cancer will survive their illness, that cancer is not contagious, and that cancer survivors have productivity rates similar to other workers.[2,36]

Categories of employment-related problems include (1) dismissal, demotion, and reduction or elimination of work-related benefits; (2) situations arising from coworkers' attitudes about cancer; and (3) problems related to survivors' attitudes about how they should be perceived by others in the workplace.[37] Discrimination can be as subtle as experiencing increased conflict with coworkers or as blatant as being terminated or rejected from a desired position.

Studies have confirmed that the work performance of cancer survivors differed little, if any, from the performance of others hired at the same age for similar assignments and that up to 80% of cancer patients returned to work after being diagnosed.[35,36,38,39] Yet an often troublesome effect of a cancer history continues to be "job-lock," where one fears leaving an undesirable position because of the potential loss of medical insurance and other benefits.[40]

Certain federal and state laws prohibit employment discrimination against qualified people with a history of cancer. Although the Federal Rehabilitation Act of 1973 is limited to those employers who receive federal funding, it can offer protection to those who qualify and feel discriminated against because of a real or perceived (by the employer) handicap.[41] Most states prohibit discrimination against the disabled in general, while a few states explicitly protect those with histories of cancer. There can be a problem, though, when the legal system attempts to label all cancer survivors as "handicapped or disabled" when there is often no visible evidence of their being either. This suggests the need for further clarification of terms through more explicit legislation.

Insurance Problems

With better access to treatment options, many cancer survivors are experiencing increased lifespans after receiving more sophisticated medical care. The availability of adequate health insurance is rarely guaranteed, and the problems created when attempting to secure or obtain these benefits can be financially and emotionally devastating. The numerous barriers to insurability include refusal of new applications, policy cancellations or reductions, higher premiums, waived or excluded preexisting conditions, and extended waiting periods.[42] These barriers may also affect the spouse or family member who carries the insurance policy. Studies suggest that 25% to 30% of cancer survivors experience some form of insurance discrimination.[42,43]

Because there is no state- or federally mandated "legal right" to health insurance, individuals should carefully examine the specific terms of their policies and the applicable state law to determine a legal violation. If an employer has more than 20 employees, it is required under COBRA, a federal law passed in 1986, to offer a continuance of group medical coverage to those whose circumstances warrant reducing or changing work hours or leaving the job.[44] The affected employee is eligible for extended coverage up to 18 months, while spouse and dependents receive these benefits for 36 months.

Other sources of assistance for insurance problems are state insurance commissions that regulate insurance rates, policy conditions, and all aspects of coverage and benefits. These state agencies are usually available to individuals with questions and complaints concerning existing policies and insurability. In addition, a number of states have introduced "high-risk pools" for those considered medically uninsurable.[45] By requiring the major insurance companies to share in the risks and expenses, more people with preexisting conditions have the opportunity to purchase comprehensive insurance plans, albeit at higher premiums. Nurses should be familiar with the available resources to assist the survivor who has employment or insurance problems. These resources are available on local, state, and national levels as described in Table 19-2.

TABLE 19-2 Local, State, and National Resources for Employment and Insurance Problems

Employment	Insurance
Local	
Disability and employment law attorneys	Insurance Department
	Social Security, local office
	Medicare
Local survivor organizations	Medicaid
	Group insurance plans
	Open enrollment periods
	Local survivor organizatons
State	
State Department of Labor, Civil Rights Division	State Insurance Commission
	"High-risk pools" (not applicable in all states)
National	
Rehabilitation Act of 1973*	COBRA (Consolidated Omnibus Budget Reconciliation Act)†
ERISA (Employee Retirement and Income Security Act)†	
National survivor organizations	National survivor organizations

*Write to Department of Justice, Civil Rights Division, Coordination and Review Section, Washington, DC 20530.

†Write to Pension and Welfare Benefits Administration, U.S. Department of Labor, Room N-5658, 200 Constitution Avenue, NW, Washington, DC 20210.

TABLE 19-3   Foci and Objectives of a Comprehensive Assessment and Intervention Program for Adult Long-Term Cancer Survivors

Focus	Specific Considerations
Physical	Follow-up potential effects of cancer and multimodal therapies Recognize endurance, fatigue, energy reserve problems based on intensity of treatment Be aware of incidence of secondary malignancy from treatment along with second or third primary tumors
Emotional	Acknowledge potential chronic anxiety associated with fear of recurrence Be alert to reactions to social stigma, changes in interpersonal relationships Be sensitive to family's adaptation to the cancer experience Acknowledge the potential existence of survivor guilt
Sexual	Consider interplay of fertility issues with coping strategies Consider intimacy needs as a subset of sexual satisfaction Discuss disclosure options relative to potential partners Anticipate concern about health of offspring
Social	Discuss concerns about friends and acquaintances and reactions to cancer history Recognize that life goals may be reprioritized Relate social adaptation to health status Encourage integration of family, friends, hobbies, and vacation into long-range plans
Vocational	Acknowledge potential job-related stress and coworkers' responses to cancer history Educate about possible discrimination at work Assist with vocational rehabilitation if necessary
Economic	Consider possible long-term financial burden Provide resources for insurance problems Encourage a balance between long- and short-term goals

SUPPORTIVE CARE

Rehabilitation Framework

In considering the options for providing support for the long-term survivor of adult cancer, the concept of rehabilitation must be addressed. Veronesi and Martino[46] stated that rehabilitation is the bridge that leads the patient from the condition of diversity to a condition of normality. Mayer[47] noted that the concept of cancer rehabilitation encompasses the theme of quality survival—not how long a person lives, but how well he or she lives within the constraints of the disease. Watson[48] described rehabilitation as an appropriate umbrella concept applicable across the entire cancer continuum. The nurse's role in cancer rehabilitation is to help the patient reduce the extent to which the cancer-related disability becomes a handicap or interferes with the ability to function in everyday life, however long that life may be. Because there is a paucity of information available on the physiologic long-term effects of cancer therapy for adults, the residual end products of therapy are unclear.[31] However, as former patients cope with extended or permanent survival, many do not return to prior levels of functioning.[49] These survivors find that they must develop strategies to cope with new situations and alterations in health status and functional abilities.

Rehabilitation in cancer care is particularly relevant, since the number of cancer survivors is predicted to increase. The growing acknowledgement of the physical, emotional, sexual, social, vocational, and economic implications of surviving cancer suggests a more aggressive approach to both assessment and intervention planning for long-term survivorship (Table 19-3). To date, interest in this subset of people with a history of cancer has been negligible and certainly not comprehensive. The systematic follow-up of former active adult patients is virtually nonexistent in the United States. This nonpractice is incompatible with a model rehabilitative approach to cancer care that includes ongoing reassessment and redefinition of goals.[50] Groenwald and Thaney[51] described rehabilitation as a dynamic process, the antithesis of customary convalescence where a person is allowed passivity while nature takes its course. Preventive and restorative goal setting become critical parameters to the enhancement of a long-term survival trajectory that is characterized by minimal debilitation and a wellness orientation. Particular attention must also be paid to the ongoing and long-range implications of financial burden imposed by cancer.[52-54]

Significant policy statements have been made by key groups that encourage future investigation into the development of rehabilitation models of cancer care. Adult cancer survivors as a subset of people facing cancer would certainly benefit by policy implementation. In 1988, Deborah Mayer and the Oncology Nursing Society coordinated an invitational conference on "Addressing Barriers to Successful Cancer Rehabilitation."[55] Three of the fifteen proposed action items specifically addressed cancer survivors and included recommendations to (1) develop a system to identify cancer survivors, (2) develop a system for long-term follow-up and monitoring of cancer survivors, and (3) identify the needs of cancer survivors.

Also in 1988, the Cancer Survivor's Bill of Rights was published by the American Cancer Society (ACS) (below). Finally, the Association of Community Cancer Centers stated that the provision of rehabilitation services to cancer patients and their families should be a basic standard of care in the community.[56] As increasing numbers of cancer patients survive, nurses can contribute to the quality and satisfaction of the survivors' lives by developing a philosophy that is both holistic and rehabilitative.[57]

American Cancer Society

THE CANCER SURVIVORS' BILL OF RIGHTS

A new population lives among us today—a new minority of 5 million people with a history of cancer. Three million of these Americans have lived with their diagnoses for five years or more.

You see these modern survivors in offices and in factories, on bicycles and cruise ships, on tennis courts, beaches and bowling alleys. You see them in all ages, shapes, sizes and colors. Usually they are unremarkable in appearance; sometimes they are remarkable for the way they have learned to live with disabilities resulting from cancer or its treatment.

Modern medical advances have returned about half of the nation's cancer patients of all ages (and 59 percent for those under the age of 55) to a normal lifespan. But the larger society has not always kept pace in helping make this lifespan truly "normal": at least, it has felt awkward in dealing with this fledgling group; at most, it has failed fully to accept survivors as functioning members.

The American Cancer Society presents this Survivors' Bill of Rights to call public attention to survivor needs, to enhance cancer care, and to bring greater satisfacton to cancer survivors, as well as to their physicians, employers, families and friends:

1. Survivors have the right to assurance of lifelong medical care, as needed. The physicians and other professionals involved in their care should continue their constant efforts to be:
● sensitive to the cancer survivors' lifestyle choices and their need for self-esteem and dignity;
● careful, no matter how long they have survived, to have symptoms taken seriously, and not have aches and pains dismissed, for fear of recurrence is a normal part of survivorship;
● informative and open, providing survivors with as much or as little candid medical information as they wish, and encouraging their informed participation in their own care;
● knowledgeable about counseling resources, and willing to refer survivors and their families as appropriate for emotional support and therapy which will improve the quality of individual lives.

2. In their personal lives, survivors, like other Americans, have the right of the pursuit of happiness. This means they have the right:
● to talk with their families and friends about their cancer experience if they wish, but to refuse to discuss it if that is their choice and not to be expected to be more upbeat or less blue than anyone else;
● to be free of the stigma of cancer as a "dread disease" in all social relations;
● to be free of blame for having gotten the disease and of guilt for having survived it;

3. In the workplace, survivors have the right to equal job opportunities. This means they have the right:
● to aspire to jobs worthy of their skills, and for which they are trained and experienced, and thus not to have to accept jobs they would not have considered before the cancer experience;
● to be hired, promoted and accepted on return to work, according to their individual abilities and qualifications, and not according to "cancer" or "disability" stereotypes;
● to privacy about their medical histories

4. Since health insurance coverage is an overriding survivorship concern, every effort should be made to assure all survivors adequate health insurance, whether public or private. This means:
● for employers, that survivors have the right to be included in group health coverage, which is usually less expensive, provides better benefits, and covers the employee regardless of health history;
● for physicians, counselors, and other professionals concerned, that they keep themselves and their survivor-clients informed and up-to-date on available group or individual health policy options, noting, for example, what major expenses like hospital costs and medical tests outside the hospital are covered and what amount must be paid before coverage (deductibles).

Resources and Interventions

Conflicting reactions to cancer survival can be a heavy burden for the strongest of individuals. Although grateful to be alive, these individuals may have difficulties adjusting to the tradeoffs of survival, that is, the possible long-term and potential unknown late effects of the disease and its treatment. As the health care profession's successes in controlling and eradicating disease increase, so too does its obligation to minimize the traumas of illness and medical interventions.

The availability of education, counseling, and supportive services becomes crucial in caring for those diagnosed with cancer. As more people live with cancer as a chronic illness, improvements in "quality of life" issues and survivor rights are a major concern. Even if support is available and adequate during the acute stage of care, an abrupt severance of this support can increase the trauma of readjusting to life as a nonhospitalized patient or cancer survivor. Although survival itself may be reward enough for some, others are seeking options to improve their current health status with hopes of preventing future problems.

From governmental agencies and medical institutions to grassroots organizations, the collective cancer survivor population is being heard as it organizes, networks, and advocates for the right to quality survival. Numerous model programs, encompassing both professional and peer support, are responding in a nationwide attempt to meet the changing needs of this growing group. However, before appropriate programs can be developed, in-depth interviews and studies must be undertaken to delineate the types of educational materials needed, the best methods for intervention, and the stages or timing to deliver information or interventions. Areas for consideration in planning interventions for long-term survivors of adult cancer include undertaking individualized needs assessments, addressing educational needs, engaging in research, and developing model programs.

Assessing individual needs

As in the acute phases of illness, it is imperative to continue assessing both the survivor's and the family's coping styles throughout the extended and permanent stages of survival. Included in this comprehensive and ongoing nursing assessment are strategies that help to resolve crisis intensity and enhance self-care. The survivor's age and developmental stage, socioeconomic background, type of cancer, prognosis, and treatment-related complications are important variables influencing his or her needs. Examples of nursing diagnoses related to an individual needs assessment include (1) ineffective patient or family coping related to ongoing surveillance for long-term effects from disease or treatment, (2) grieving related to loss of job after successful treatment for cancer, (3) alteration in sexuality related to difficulties in establishing intimate relationships, and (4) knowledge deficit related to the recognition of cancer recurrence symptomatology.

Addressing educational needs related to survivorship

During the development of educational resources for survivors, nurses must continue to acknowledge the different needs and information preferences of individuals and families. Researchers at Stanford University found that patients want to be well informed about potential or expected problems.[58] Individuals who seek much information may request specifics about cancer recurrence or anticipated problems relative to their diagnosis. Since fear of recurrence and worries about health are common among survivors, nurses can help reduce the stress associated with the unknown by anticipating crises points and sharing this information with survivors. Examples of time-related crises that may be experienced by survivors are anniversaries of diagnosis and treatment cessation, birthdays, holidays, yearly examinations, and waiting for the 5-year survival mark. Situation-specific crises include diagnosis disclosure to friends and coworkers, hearing stories about cancer, waiting for results of follow-up examinations, symptomatology assessment, revealing past medical history, and establishing intimate relationships. If a crisis becomes unmanageable or persistent, nursing referrals can be made for an appropriate intervention.

Survivors and their families may want to know about potential secondary benefits of the cancer experience.[46] These benefits, frequently emphasized by survivors themselves, may include a new-found zest for life, value reprioritization, and a greater sense of generalized well-being.

Promotion of a greater awareness of cancer survivorship issues should begin during basic nursing education. To sensitize student nurses to the continuing need for supportive care, interactions with long-term survivors are recommended.[47]

Engaging in research

Although the psychosocial ramifications were the first to be studied, relatively little systematic and longitudinal information on coping from diagnosis through "cure" has been obtained.[5] What is currently needed is a comprehensive assessment format to study the long-term needs of adult survivors, that is, a format similar to those available for studying children.[59] Areas for research include (1) the relationship of developmental stage to psychosocial sequelae, (2) description of survival trajectories, (3) family dilemmas during long-term survivorship, (4) the interrelationship of physical compromise and coping problems, (5) identification of the mediators of stress throughout survivorship, (6) association of the attitudes of the health care team with recurrence anxiety, and (7) how time influences fears of relapse.[29,31,57]

Developing model programs

Once survivor-specific assessments identify areas of individual need, a more general assessment of community resources already available for cancer survivors can then be performed. These two steps would logically precede the development of any formal survivor program. Including survivors themselves in dialogues concerning the planning and implementation of these programs will enhance program development and reliability. A variety of support options, whether individual or group related, allows one to better tailor interventions to the survivor's needs.

The success of any cancer survivor program will depend on (1) the commitment of the health care team to provide ongoing evaluation and planning for change as the subject lives with a history of cancer, (2) the identification of key individuals to coordinate activities within and among team members, (3) the involvement of the patient and family in the program from initial diagnosis, and (4) the effectiveness of communication among team members.[60] This approach encourages the early recognition of problems during therapy that is imperative for the possible prevention of long-term sequelae.[61]

The majority of long-term survivor programs are non–hospital-based programs and include national and local cancer hotlines, regional chapters of national organizations, and community networks that focus on peer support. The National Coalition for Cancer Survivorship (NCCS) (323 Eighth Street, SW, Albuquerque, NM 87102 [505]764-9956) serves as a resource to network individuals and groups concerned with cancer survivorship issues and has increased access to information, referrals, resources, educational opportunities, and professional and peer support. Refer to the Yellow Pages of this text for an extended list of resources.

Hospital- or community-based survivor programs can have multiple components. Comprehensive follow-up clinics provide surveillance for physical and psychological long-term effects. These clinics can be wellness-oriented, emphasizing the importance of proper nutrition, the need for individualized exercise programs, and disease-prevention behaviors. Another component can help to clarify misconceptions about cancer and address survivor limitations by providing information about cancer survival to coworkers and employers. This information should be provided by the treatment team before the survivor returns to the workplace. Some programs offer survivor reunions within hospitals or the community at large. Included in these reunions are those who continue to live with a history of cancer, their families and friends, and their health care providers.

All these options and approaches for long-term survivor program development become particularly important in light of the growing number of survivors. Programs must deal with all developmental stages, ranging from the elderly[32] to the growing number of younger adult survivors.

CONCLUSION

Long-term survivorship of adult cancers has many psychosocial ramifications. The definitions of survivorship, the concept of survivorship as a continuum, major psychosocial themes, employment and insurance discrimination, rehabilitation framework, and resources and interventions have been discussed.

Rosetta Poletti,[62] in her address to the Second European Conference on Clinical Oncology and Cancer Nursing, stated that "The goal of cancer nursing should be to assist the person to be a fully functioning person first and a cancer patient second." Within a framework of rehabilitation, support programs for cancer survivors can be developed in partnership with health care professionals and survivors and focus on delivering optimal care during all stages of survival. Nursing, with its dynamic, holistic focus, is in an ideal position to promote cancer survivor rehabilitation.

• • •

Funded in part by NIHCA 23074 and Arizona Disease Control Research Commission 33640000000-1-1-AP-6621.

REFERENCES

1. Cella DF, Lesko LM: Cancer survivors: Watch for signs of stress even years later. Oncology Rounds (Primary Care and Cancer), Burroughs-Welcome Co, 1988, pp 1-9.
2. American Cancer Society: Cancer Facts and Figures. Atlanta, Ga, The Society, 1988.
3. National Cancer Institute: Surveillance, Epidemiology, and End Results Program (SEER), Annual Cancer Statistics Review. Bethesda, Md, The Institute, November 1984.
4. Fobair P, Mages NL: Psychosocial morbidity among cancer patient survivors, in Ahmed P (ed): Coping With Cancer. New York, Elsevier, 1981, pp 285-308.
5. Cella DF: Cancer survival: Psychosocial and public issues. Cancer Invest 5:59-67, 1987.
6. Fobair P, Hoppe RT, Bloom J, et al: Psychosocial problems among survivors of Hodgkin's disease. J Clin Oncol 4:805-814, 1986.
7. Goldberg RJ, Tull RM: The Psychosocial Dimensions of Cancer. New York, The Free Press, 1983, pp 40-80.
8. Mish FC (ed): Webster's Ninth New Collegiate Dictionary. Springfield, Mass, Merriam-Webster, 1983.
9. Hammond GD: The cure of childhood cancers. Cancer 58:407-413, 1986.
10. Holland J: Psychological aspects of oncology. Med Clin North Am 61:737-748, 1977.
11. Roud PC: Psychosocial variables associated with the exceptional survival of patients with advanced malignant disease. J Natl Med Assoc 79:97-102, 1987.
12. Vought CA, Dintruff DL, Fotopoulos SS: Adaptations to the constraints of cancer: Motivational issues, in Ahmed P (ed): Living and Dying with Cancer. New York, Elsevier, 1981, pp 205-219.
13. Fobair P: A review of Smith K, Lesko L: Psychosocial problems in cancer survivors. Oncology 2:41-44, 1988.
14. Mullan F: Seasons of survival: Reflections of a physician with cancer. N Engl J Med 313:270-273, 1985.
15. Weddington WW, Segraves KB, Simon MA: Current and lifetime incidence of psychiatric disorders among a group of extremity sarcoma survivors. J Psychosom Res 30:121-125, 1986.

16. Shanfield SB: On surviving cancer: Psychological considerations. Comprehensive Psych 21:128-134, 1980.

17. Chang PN, Nesbit ME, Youngren N, et al: Personality characteristics and psychosocial adjustment of long-term survivors of childhood cancer. J Psychosoc Oncol 5:43-58, 1987.

18. Tebbi CK, Mallon JC: Long-term psychosocial outcome among cancer amputees in adolescence and early adulthood. J Psychosoc Oncol 5:69-82, 1987.

19. Schmale AH, Morrow GR, Schmitt MH, et al: Well-being of cancer survivors. Psychosom Med 45:163-169, 1983.

20. Smith K, Lesko LM: Psychosocial problems in cancer survivors. Oncology 2:33-44, 1988.

21. Gotay CC: Quality of life among survivors of childhood cancer: A critical review and implications for intervention. J Psychosoc Oncol 5:5-23, 1987.

22. Woods NF, Earp JL: Women with cured breast cancer: A study of mastectomy patients in North Carolina. Nurs Res 27:279-285, 1978.

23. Rieker PP, Edbril SD, Garnick MB: Curative testis cancer therapy: Psychosocial sequelae. J Clin Oncol 3:1117-1126, 1985.

24. Cella DF, Tross S: Psychological adjustment to survival from Hodgkin's disease. J Consult Clin Psychol 54:616-622, 1986.

25. Mullan F: Re-entry: the educational needs of the cancer survivor. Health Educ Q 10:88-94, 1984 (suppl).

26. Maher EL: Anomic aspects of recovery from cancer. Soc Sci Med 16:907-912, 1982.

27. Northouse LL: Mastectomy patients and the fear of cancer recurrence. Cancer Nurs 4:213-220, 1981.

28. Welch-McCaffrey D: Cancer anxiety and quality of life. Cancer Nurs 8:151-158, 1985.

29. Quigley KM: The adult cancer survivor: Psychosocial consequences of cure. Semin Oncol Nurs 5:63-69, 1989.

30. Gorsynski JG, Holland JC: Psychological aspects of testicular cancer. Semin Oncol 6:125-129, 1979.

31. Loescher LJ, Welch-McCaffrey D, Leigh SA, et al: Surviving Adult Cancers. I. Physiologic effects. Ann Intern Med 3:411-432, 1989; II. Psychosocial sequelae. Ann Intern Med 3:517-524, 1989.

32. Welch-McCaffrey D: Family issues in cancer care: Current dilemmas—future directions. J Psychosoc Oncol 6:199-211, 1988.

33. Hoffman B: Employment discrimination based on cancer history: The need for federal legislation. Temple Law Q 59:4-9, 1986.

34. Wasserman AL, Thompson ET, Wilmas A, et al: The psychosocial status of survivors of childhood/adolescent Hodgkin's disease. Am J Dis Child 141:626-631, 1987.

35. Crothers HM: Employment problems of cancer survivors: Local problems and local solutions, in Proceedings of the Workshop on Employment, Insurance and the Patient with Cancer. New Orleans, American Cancer Society, 1986, pp 51-57.

36. Wheatley GM, Cunnick WR, Wright BP, et al: Employment of persons with a history of treatment for cancer. Cancer 33:441-445, 1974.

37. Feldman F: Female cancer patients and caregivers: Experiences in the workplace, in Stellman S (ed): Women and Cancer. New York, Harrington Park Press, 1987, pp 137-153.

38. Stone RW: Employing the recovered cancer patient. Cancer 36:285-286, 1975.

39. Mellette SJ: The cancer patient at work. ACS Prof Ed Publ 35:6-8, 1985.

40. Greenleigh Associates: Report on the social, economic, and psychological needs of cancer patients in California, in proceedings of Western States Conference on Cancer Rehabilitation. Palo Alto, Calif, Bull Publishing Co, March 1982.

41. Rehabilitation Act of 1973. 29 U.S.C. (United States Code) 701 *et seq.*

42. Crothers H: Health insurance: Problems and solutions for people with cancer histories, in Proceedings of the 5th National Conference on Human Values and Cancer. San Francisco, American Cancer Society, 1987, pp 100-109.

43. Burton L, Zones J: The incidence of insurance barriers and employment discrimination among Californians with a cancer health history in 1983: A projection. Los Angeles, American Cancer Society (Calif division), 1982.

44. Consolidated Omnibus Budget Reconciliation Act (COBRA). 1986, 42 U.S.C. 300 bb *et seq.*

45. Trippler A: Comprehensive health insurance for high risk individuals: A state by state analysis. Fergus Falls, MN: Communicating for Agriculture, 1987.

46. Veronesi U, Martino G: Can life be the same after cancer treatment? Tumori 64:345-351, 1978.

47. Mayer NH: Concepts in cancer rehabilitation. Semin Oncol 2:393-398, 1975.

48. Watson PG: Rehabilitation philosophy: A means of fostering a positive attitude toward cancer. J Enterostom Ther 13:153-156, 1986.

49. Kudsk EG, Hoffman GS: Rehabilitation of the cancer patient. Primary Care 14:381-390, 1987.

50. Habeck RV, Romsaas EP, Olsen SJ: Cancer rehabilitation and continuing care: A case study. Cancer Nurs 7:315-320, 1984.

51. Groenwald SL, Thaney K: Rehabilitation, in Groenwald SL (ed): Cancer Nursing: Principles and Practice. Boston, Jones and Bartlett, 1987, pp 749-758.

52. Houts PS, Harvey HA, Simmonds MA, et al: Characteristics of patients at risk for financial burden because of cancer and its treatment. J Psychosoc Oncol 3:15-22, 1985.

53. McNaull FW: The costs of cancer: A challenge to health care providers. Cancer Nurs 4:207-212, 1981.

54. Baird SB: Economic realities in the treatment and care of the cancer patient. Topics Clin Nurs 2:67-80, 1981.

55. Mayer D: An invitational conference addressing barriers to successful cancer rehabilitation, in Proceedings of the 1988 Oncology Nursing Society President's Grant, Boston, August 1988.

56. Enck RE: ACCC standards: Past, present and future. J Cancer Progr Management 2:11-20, 1987.

57. Dudas S, Carlson CE: Cancer rehabilitation. Oncol Nurs Forum 15:183-188, 1988.

58. Fobair P, Hoppe R, Bloom J, et al: Psychosocial problems among survivors of Hodgkin's disease. J Clin Oncol 4:805-814, 1986.

59. Fergusson J, Ruccione K, Wasderwitz M, et al: Time required to assess children for the late effects of treatment. Cancer Nurs 10:300-310, 1987.

60. Broadwell DC: Rehabilitation needs of the patient with cancer. Cancer 60:563-568, 1987.

61. Andersen BL: Sexual functioning morbidity among cancer survivors. Cancer 55:1835-1842, 1985.

62. Poletti R: Living a full life with cancer, in Proceedings of the Second European Conference on Clinical Oncology and Cancer Nursing. Amsterdam, ECCO, November 1983.